LINCOLN CHRISTIAN COLLEGE AND SEMINARY

JJ0660488

Laughing
in the Face
of AIDS

The Authors

Dr. G. Edward Rozar, Jr., a former thoracic surgeon, now serves as director of a laboratory in Marshfield, Wisconsin. One of the first infected medical personnel to "go public," Dr. Rozar is active in the AIDS awareness effort, speaking across the country, through the media, and before Congress.

Co-author David B. Biebel is editor of *Physician*, a publication of Focus on the Family.

Laughing in the Face of AIDS

A Surgeon's Personal Battle

G. Edward Rozar, Jr., M.D.

with

David B. Biebel

Foreword by W. Shepherd Smith

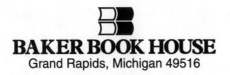

BAKER BOOK HOUSE
Grand Rapids, Michigan 49516

Copyright 1992 by G. Edward Rozar, Jr.

Library of Congress Cataloging-in-Publication Data
Rozar, G. Edward Jr.
　　Laughing in the face of AIDS : a surgeon's personal battle / G.
Edward Rozar with David B. Biebel.
　　　　p.　　cm.
　　Includes bibliographical references.
　　ISBN 0-8010-7767-2 (cloth).—ISBN 0-8010-7765-6 (pbk.)
　　1. Rozar, G. Edward—Health. 2. AIDS (Disease)—United States—
Biography. 3. Surgeons—United States—Biography. 4. AIDS (Disease)—
Religious aspects—Christianity. I. Biebel, David B. II. Title.
　　RC607.A26R68　1992
　　362.1'96972'0092—dc20
　　[B]　　　　　　　　　　　　　　　　　　　　　　　　92-12924

Printed in the United States of America

Scripture references not otherwise marked are from the New American Standard
Bible. Copyright © 1960, 1962, 1963, 1968, 1971, 1972, 1973, 1975, 1977 by
the Lockman Foundation.

Some references are from the New International Version (NIV), © 1973, 1978,
1984 by the International Bible Society.

Then they cried out to the LORD in their trouble;
He saved them out of their distresses.
He sent His word and healed them,
And delivered *them* from their destructions.
Psalm 107:19–20

This book is dedicated to

my lovely wife, Donna;

our five beautiful children:

Jonathan Edward

Victoria Kay

Jonathan Wayne

David Michael

Christina Michelle

Pastor Ed Gungor of Believers' Church

Glenn Klein

and Jesus Christ,

my Healer and Lord.

97217

Contents

Foreword

For many years the church in America has felt itself immune from HIV, the virus that causes AIDS. Few people believed AIDS would ever enter the church, let alone infect godly people. We now know such thinking was truly wishful, part of our human nature to deny that such tragedies can touch us or our friends.

Although we may understand that the church will not remain untouched by AIDS, we still have a host of concerns and questions. What should we do when a family member becomes infected? How should a congregation respond to an infected member? What would God have us do in the age of AIDS?

Ed Rozar has acquired HIV. I know Ed personally and can attest to the fact that he is truly a godly man who loves his Lord. His genial countenance, caring nature, and spiritual character have allowed him to laugh in the face of AIDS. As you come to know Ed through these pages, you will realize that only the power given by God allows for such courage and strength. Ed's story offers inspiration and hope to those enduring hardship. But more than that, it helps answer some of our questions about how we should respond to AIDS/HIV.

Laughing in the Face of AIDS gives us insight not only into the power of God but also into the goodness of humans. With remarkable courage Ed shares both the highs and the lows. Because of Ed's intense honesty, the book speaks to our hearts in ways few books do.

So this is not as much a book about AIDS as it is a book about life. You will read about struggles common to all of us, as well as many joys and accomplishments. Although the book teaches several lessons, I'd like to highlight three powerful themes.

First, it illustrates the power of God in the face of adversity. And when I say adversity, I do not mean that lightly. Ed is the father of five lively children. Nearing the peak of his career, Ed had virtually everything taken from him. Yet he was able to realize how much more he was given.

Second, it calls us to examine our relationships with our own family members. What are our priorities? How do we respond to those who depend on us? Do we truly share our love with them?

Third, it challenges us as Christians to respond to the AIDS epidemic as Christ would have us. We are summoned to think more seriously about a disease that has entered the church and is spreading relentlessly across America, a disease that can no longer be ignored by the body of Christ.

God has equipped Ed Rozar to be an excellent spokesman for this mission. Ed is a child of God whose obedience humbles us. Ed is a father whose love of family inspires us. Ed is a doctor whose medical advice with respect to AIDS instructs us. Ed clearly points out the challenge AIDS poses and then gently with love takes away our fears and gives us courage to face this growing epidemic.

When we began Americans for a Sound AIDS/HIV Policy in 1987, it was our hope that we would never have to meet an Ed Rozar. Today I understand the critical role that Ed and others like him play in instructing us, chastening us, and guiding us to follow Christ's example in the face of this deadly foe. I thank God for bringing Ed into my life.

W. Shepherd Smith, Jr.
President
Americans for a Sound AIDS/HIV Policy

Introduction

The journey you are about to embark on reveals how awesome God's grace is. As you travel along with me in this book, I hope you will be encouraged by my transition from shattered dreams to wholeness. Our family is looking forward to the future. Perhaps your view of the future will be enlightened also.

I want to thank especially Dave Biebel for putting this material together. He has invested two years of work which included hours of audio taping, and sifting through 700 pages of typewritten material. Without his dedicated efforts my story would not be in print.

Baker Book House encouraged and helped throughout the process of writing and editing the manuscript.

The people of Believers' Church in Marshfield supported us as we opened our hearts and lives to public scrutiny. Without their encouragement and prayers, the energy necessary to complete this project would not have been available. Pastors Ed Gungor, Glenn Smith, and Randy Burkhart have been instrumental in cheering me and the family along this journey. Glenn Klein and Jerry Dahlke continue to be there for me in times of need and rejoicing.

I cannot possibly mention all the people praying for us. Christians from all walks of life have taken us under wing and cared for us. The Marshfield Clinic has taken complete responsibility for my health care and continued employment.

There is no turning back, life goes on; God alone is faithful and just.

G. Edward Rozar, Jr., M.D.

⊿ 1 ⊾

Heart to Heart

*a*s a heart surgeon, I knew that having your heart stopped by somebody you didn't know, to make repairs you needed but didn't understand, was nobody's idea of a good time. So quite often I would sit on my patient's bed, get out a felt-tip pen and sketch on the sheets what I was going to do in the operating room.

"You'll get in trouble drawing on those sheets," the patient would protest, intently studying my artwork.

"No," I laughed, "they won't kick me off the staff!"

If the patient needed one or more bypasses, I would diagram the heart and its major vessels, and show where the particular blockages were. Then I would show how we would create conduits around those obstructions, so the heart could get the blood supply it needed.

You could almost see a light going on, especially if no other doctor had taken the time to explain the procedure. That light was partly from the patient's new understanding, but it was also because our new relationship had transformed a clinical procedure into a personal experience we would both share.

I was a good heart surgeon, with good results. But I always leveled with my patients; the risk is never zero percent. Even if their surgery was more "routine," with a risk of only 1 or 2 percent, I still made it clear that to make that statistic, one or two out of a hundred patients failed to survive.

Not that I wanted to scare anybody. I wanted them to know that as far as I was concerned, every patient was unique. You can never say that even 1 percent is a low number, as if it doesn't mean anything. It means something to somebody. In fact, it means *everything* to somebody. Because 1 percent is 100 percent if it's you, it's never right to pretend that statistics like these represent anything other than real people with real and sometimes excruciating personal needs. When any of my patients didn't make it, there was a void that couldn't be filled by any other human being.

Another reason I tried to befriend my patients before we went into surgery was that I knew it was then or maybe never. As with children growing up, the time to establish that bond of trust is before the storm occurs—whether the crisis is because of illness, accident, or just the fact that adolescence has rendered them temporarily impaired.

Sometimes, even when we did the best we could surgically in our first attempt, patients would develop complications requiring us to go in again. It was always easier to sit down with these patients and their families and explain something as unwelcome as this (to us, as well as to them) if the foundation had been laid earlier. Because they knew I cared for them, not only did they believe me enough to put their lives very literally in my hands again, but they were able to approach our setback with confidence and hope.

I loved cardiac surgery. I loved the challenge. It was the peak I climbed to through thirteen years of surgical experience and training after medical school. Most of all, I loved helping patients who would have died otherwise. And I was always glad to have a heart-to-heart talk with them before it was time for me to reach for the knife.

Now that I've put the scalpel down, I want to have a heart-to-heart talk with you about infection with HIV (the virus that causes AIDS). HIV is the reason I'm not operating today. Somewhere along the line, on an unknown day—probably during surgery—I became infected. Now that I know what it feels like to be a patient as well as a physician, perhaps our chat will be even more eye to eye and heart to heart than we could have had before.

Maybe you are HIV-infected, and that is the reason you're reading this. More likely, you are not. You may not even know anybody who has this disease. But if things go the way I expect, you will in the near future, and it probably will surprise you who it is. So now is a good time to prepare yourself.

If you're like I was when I got my own diagnosis, you don't really know very much about HIV infection. I'll try to answer the questions (at least most of them) that are banging around in your mind.

You can trust me as we look at this complicated disease, though you may not always agree with my conclusions. Unlike some parties involved, I don't come to it with any political, personal, or professional agendas. All I really care about is that you hear the truth about AIDS. Much more importantly, that you come to know the Truth (that's what Jesus called himself) who is able to set us free to live and to laugh, even in the face of a diagnosis as devastating as AIDS.

There was a time when my attitude toward persons with AIDS was different from what it is today. Not that I was as judgmental as some people have been, but neither was I convinced that health-care workers (specifically, myself) should risk doing procedures that seemed unnecessary. For instance, when I was at West Virginia University as an assistant professor, we were asked to do a lung biopsy on a person obviously afflicted with *pneumocystis carinii,* a rare pneumonia that is one of the signs of AIDS. I was thinking, "Maybe it'll go away, so I don't have to put myself at risk." Little did I know that I was already HIV-infected myself.

As a Christian and a doctor, my experience with the diagnosis and treatment of my own disease has helped me see beyond statistics and symptoms to the needs of AIDS patients and their families. To convince you that I know what I'm talking about, I'll risk telling you more than you may care to hear concerning our personal, marital, and family journey with this modern-day plague.

Right from the start, I want to be clear about why I've written this book. I want to achieve one thing and avoid another. First let me say that I don't want your pity—though I must confess it feels good sometimes. As far as I'm concerned, I'm not an "innocent victim." Although I got this disease from an unidentified patient, that was part of the risk associated with my choosing to become a surgeon. Not that I would ever make light of that career. It was everything I wanted and more, maybe too much so. But I'm getting ahead of myself. When this story is over, I want you to know Ed Rozar as more than a born-again evangelical HIV-positive cardiac surgeon.

In terms of what I hope to achieve, I want to give you a deeper knowledge of what HIV is. I also want you to see what HIV can do to its carriers as well as to the people who know and love them. But this whole effort will have been wasted if I fail to convince you to stop and get in touch with the Lord. I'm confident he will show you creative ways to touch the lives of (us) modern-day lepers, just as he touched the lepers of his own day. Then, whether you're the one who's hurting or the one who wants to help, you may discover something truly remarkable that applies to any difficulty, affliction, loss, or sorrow conceivable this side of heaven—that his healing power can transform weakness into strength, darkness into light, sorrow into joy, and sickness into health.

Since our situation became public, we've had many opportunities to address the issues of AIDS. Donna and I have appeared on NBC's "Today" show, CBS's "This Morning," ABC's "20/20," CBN's "700 Club," and been featured in a multitude of other TV, radio, and newspaper interviews. I have participated in several public forums, and testified before Congress in relation to the "Kimberly Bergalis" bill. I plan to take you behind the scenes of some of those situations in the coming pages.

When I look back over all of those experiences, and anticipate those that lie ahead, three things hit me. First, many people, especially politicians and some physicians, don't show much common sense when it comes to AIDS policy. Second, if I'm accurately hearing people in the lay audiences I address, the public is clearly not going to stand for pretense and deception much longer. In my mind, what is sometimes labeled "hysteria" is the result of reasonable people demanding what's right.

Third, not everyone is happy when I mix Christianity with what they consider a purely medical issue. This doesn't bother me much, though, since it is *because of my experience with HIV infection* that my faith has become such an integral part of who I am today. I couldn't separate who I am from what I believe at this point, even if I tried. Besides, is it not more than a little hypocritical for people who have turned a clearly public-health issue into a matter of civil rights to accuse me of mixing issues?

I have had many opportunities to address different groups. When I do, there are several questions I hear repeatedly. The school kids want to know about Magic Johnson, safe sex, and condoms. Parents are desperate to keep their kids from getting AIDS through promiscuity. (Or are they more afraid that they themselves may get it?) Some people wonder if they can become HIV-infected through casual contact; for instance, from public toilets, shared utensils, mosquito bites. One person even asked me if he might get AIDS from taking prescription pills.

Increasingly, public-policy issues are brought up by both professional and lay audiences. Should there be mandatory testing of health-care workers (and/or patients)? Could the whole problem be solved if everybody was tested and those who tested positive were quarantined somewhere?

In church settings, it's not too difficult to sense unexpressed opinions, the most common of which might be: AIDS only happens to bad people. So why are you bothering us with this? We're not at risk. It's *their* problem, not ours, and it probably serves them right. Nobody in my family, or even any of my friends, has it. So let the government take care of it; I have more important things to think about.

Usually toward the very end of any meeting I address, somebody will have the courage to verbalize what everybody has been thinking the whole time: "Are you and your wife still having sex? Is she HIV-positive, too?"

Occasionally, I hear the question I love to answer: "How do you keep going—loving, living, laughing—in the face of something as terrifying as AIDS?"

In the pages that follow, I'll try to answer these and other questions. In a sense, it's as close as I can come to sitting down and having a heart-to-heart talk with you about all these things.

In a large audience, there will often be people who are really struggling. I can see it in their eyes. It may be AIDS, or it may be cancer. Perhaps infidelity or divorce or another personal loss has broken their hearts and they're groping for a little hope in their quiet desperation. These are the people I look for now, though I doubt I could have connected as personally with their pain before my own experience with this disease. They're really all around us, inside the church and especially outside—people searching for someone to believe, and a reason to carry on.

Maybe you're one of those hurting people. You've picked up this book (or somebody's given it to you), but you've been so down for so long you're afraid to believe that what you long for is really possible. It is! Peace, serenity, reconciliation, wholeness, even joy—these are all possible even in the face of AIDS. Despite this illness, life is better for me now than it ever was before.

I invite you to journey with me a little while, in the hope that as we walk together you'll see, as I have, that beyond the sometimes excruciating losses of life there is more, perhaps more than we could have known unless things of lesser importance had been stripped away.

The apostle Paul—who knew a lot about both suffering and joy—penned some words nearly two thousand years ago that are as inspiring today as they were then: "Therefore we do not lose heart, but though our outer man is decaying, yet our inner man is being renewed day by day. For momentary, light affliction is producing for us an eternal weight of glory far beyond all comparison, while we look not at the things which are seen, but at the things which are not seen; for the things which are seen are temporal, but the things which are not seen are eternal" (2 Cor. 4: 16–18).

Without doubt, before the diagnosis of my HIV infection turned life upside down for the Rozar clan, words like these made sense on one level. I believed in God and his Word and had been a born-again Christian since 1974. So I knew Paul's thoughts were certainly true and worth contemplating. But, in another way that is hard to explain precisely, I don't think this passage and others like it had penetrated much below the surface of my mind and reached my heart.

For now, maybe it's enough to say that the things that were "seen"—for a cardiac surgeon, there can be many of these, not all of them bad, either—seemed real enough and well worth investing in. The unseen, eternal things seemed to be for another time and place—specifically, later, maybe as late as when I would see the Lord face to face.

Whether my perspective and priorities got turned upside down or inside out as the result of my diagnosis, I can't quite tell for sure. I do know that it was because of this illness, not in spite of it, that God's Word, in fact, God himself, has become more real than anything I have ever known before. My hope is that you will experience this renewal, too, even if you're not grappling with something as dreadful as AIDS.

Sometimes when reading books like this, or hearing speakers describe their victories of faith, it's tempting to think that what worked for them is great, but it could never apply to you because your own faith seems so deficient by comparison. But here's a little secret: The saints of God were all sinners (a lot like you and me) who were willing to allow his Spirit to renew and empower their own.

Throughout the Bible are stories of sinners transformed into powerful spokespersons for God, but there are no saints who were magically modified as if by the stroke of some celestial magic wand. No matter who you are, no matter what you've done, no matter how old or how young you may be, and whatever your health is now, God loves you and has in his mind a destiny for you that is more magnificent than you could ever imagine in your wildest dreams.

What I'm trying to say is that God uses real people, just like you and me. To prove that, I will let my life become an open book, dog-eared and torn pages and all, in hopes that when all is said and done, you will be encouraged, strengthened, and better equipped to run the specific race and finish the uniquely designed course that is stretching out before you.

2

Parables and Realities

As early as I can recall, I learned about the Garden of Eden, Adam and Eve, and Noah's Ark. After all, I grew up in the church, went to Sunday school, catechism classes, confirmation—the works. Basically, though, I was just going through the motions. As far as I was concerned, stories like these were parables to teach us something, but I wasn't quite sure what for a long, long time.

Why drag the Garden of Eden and Noah's Ark into a book about AIDS? For a couple of good reasons, but I don't want to spill all the beans right now. I will say this much, however: If you want to understand how such an infernal disease could even exist, you have to go all the way back to the Garden.

If you want to see how something invisible—almost a quarter million HIV viruses will fit within the period at the end of this sentence—could threaten whole nations (as it now does in Africa) or even the whole world, just read the first few pages of Genesis. Didn't Noah's Ark save the human race from a worldwide disaster similar to what we have with

AIDS—a multifaceted global catastrophe, the impact of which no one could escape?

In my wildest nightmares, I never imagined I would become infected with HIV, the modern plague. For one thing, I was never sick, at least until 1985—and even for some time after that I felt healthy as a horse. After all, health and strength are basic requirements if you want to be a cardiac surgeon. Besides, growing up in a traditional home long before AIDS was ever heard of, I figured bad things happen mainly to bad people. Compared to the criminals I often heard about, we were pretty good people. My father was a lawyer. My mother was a schoolteacher with two Master's degrees. They were both quite strict and always right, a serious problem for a precocious youngster who figured he was right all the time, too.

As a boy I spent much energy trying to please my father, but sometimes ended up in no-win situations. Once, when chemicals killed part of our lawn, I became the prime suspect. Dad wouldn't take "I don't know how it happened" for an answer. If I didn't "tell the truth," he said, I was going to regret it. Finally, in desperation, I lied to appease him, then took the consequences just to get off the witness stand.

For some reason, I didn't end up resenting Dad as much as I might have. I don't have bitter feelings about him. As far as I can tell, I've forgiven him. The more I learn about fathering, the more I conclude that he probably didn't have a very good role model himself. But I have to agree with people who point out how much more difficult it is to develop a close, loving relationship with your heavenly Father if you have not experienced something similar with your earthly father.

Another negative result of my strict upbringing was inner conflict, especially the sense of rebellion, I had throughout adolescence. It was always my goal to become a physician, since that was what Dad wanted me to be. To express some kind of independence—as teens often do—I took up smoking and got involved with some other crazy stuff it wouldn't edify you to hear about.

I managed to concentrate enough on my studies in high school to graduate a year early and immediately entered college in the summer of 1966. Despite my continuing rebellious attitudes, I was intelligent enough to make very good grades my first two and a half years at the University of Georgia and get accepted by the Medical College of Georgia.

After being accepted into med school, my academics went on cruise control. All that driving and striving had finally paid off, but I decompressed so much that I almost didn't graduate from college. In fact, I had to go to summer school to raise my grade in biochemistry from an F to an A. I sowed even wilder oats during that period, increasing my smoking to two packs a day and my alcohol consumption to a level where it still amazes me I didn't end up killing myself or somebody else. Once, when I was driving drunk, we ran off the road right on campus; I bent the car's frame, but nobody was hurt. Another time when I was in the same condition, I ran a stop sign and just missed hitting a police officer, without even getting a ticket.

Looking back at that period, I wonder sometimes at the way I was protected from my own stupidity. It wasn't luck, I'm sure. I don't believe in luck, good or bad. Obviously, God had something else planned for me. Though I didn't know it at the time, my life and destiny were in his hands. Not that I wanted much to do with that notion. Why drag ideas like dependence and submission into the mind and heart of someone so obviously headed for success?

Nonetheless, there was one guy on campus, a Campus Crusade for Christ representative, who really got under my skin. Their first "spiritual law," about God loving me and having a wonderful plan for my life, just didn't compute, in more ways than one. I certainly didn't want to hear anything about law number two, that my own sin had separated me from God and made it impossible for me to know and experience either his love or his plan.

This fellow never gave up on me, although I mocked him relentlessly, harassed him without mercy, and continually made him the object of practical jokes. Once we even toilet-papered his dorm room. But no matter how hard I tried to ignore him, there was something about his life and something about his message that I just couldn't evade. Perhaps in my deepest self I was afraid he was right. There *was* something missing in my life, but at that point I wasn't quite ready to find out from anyone what it was. I would just figure it out myself, as I had done with everything of importance before that.

When I was a sophomore at the Medical College of Georgia, I did attend church once or twice. I'm not sure to this day why. The pastor even came out to visit, but we didn't talk much about spiritual things. Perhaps he figured I was already a believer, or else I managed to derail such discussions.

Anyhow, I sailed through medical school without much trouble, graduating in 1973. I began my internship in a small surgical program in Norfolk, Virginia, mainly because I wanted to get out of Georgia and away from home. It was time to move on, establish my own identity, live my own life.

That same summer, I met Donna Mummau, a nurse practitioner at the hospital where I was a house officer. One day I was studying in the library, and she just came over and asked my name. I had been dating a little, but Donna and I started going out together, and we've been together ever since. This, I suppose, is one of the more amazing facts of my life, since in some ways Donna and I were very different, while in other ways we were so painfully alike.

For instance, although I've always been pro-life (and we both are, now), at that point Donna was outspokenly pro-abortion. Resolving differences like that might have been easier if we hadn't both been such independent and opinionated folks who never backed down. Illogical as it may sound, after verbally fighting it out a few dozen times, we finally concluded we should either leave each other alone or get married. In 1974, we chose the latter.

It didn't take long, though, to discover that getting married hadn't erased the ego in either of us. All it took was a bad decision, one of the worst we've ever made: We bought an old house with the specific goal of redoing the whole thing. We didn't know any better, but with me a perfectionist surgeon-type and Donna a strong-willed independent woman, the sparks were flying right from the start.

Wallpapering together was a lot like mud wrestling. Stripping the walls wasn't so bad. It was messy enough, but we managed okay. Although we'd heard that couples should never wallpaper together, being the kind of people we are, we had to learn why the hard way.

As a surgical resident who spent so much time in the operating room, my mind-set was: "If it's worth doing, do it right—*exactly* right." Perfection was not to be the exception, but the rule. My compulsivity wasn't inherent or pathological; it was cultivated. When it came to matching wallpaper edges, as far as I was concerned, there was only one way to do that, too—the right way (*my* way). But Donna, not being mechanically inclined, didn't need to have it as precisely "right" as I did. The result was that we could never agree that a room, or even part of a room, was satisfactory until we had haggled over it and worked on it to the point of exhaustion.

We solved the problem not by finding a way to cooperate, but by devising ways to finish portions of the job without the other party's involvement. For instance, Donna and a girlfriend papered one of the rooms while I was working. I recall inspecting it with mixed feelings. I was glad it was done, even if it didn't look quite right.

Just so you know how intense I really was, while Donna was in Charlottesville for a weekend, I redid the whole kitchen by myself—tore out the floor, cabinets, and sink, and rebuilt it all before she came home. I stayed up all night to finish, but I was used to staying up all night, so that was no big deal.

We really had some difficulties in those early years. A surgical residency is tough enough on a marriage, without trying to restore an old house in your spare time. It's amazing that we stayed together; in fact, we alternated between fighting tooth and nail and giving each other the silent treatment.

Old-fashioned as it may sound, the reason we made it was our shared commitment that divorce was not an acceptable option. We were in this for the duration, "Come hell or high water," as my daddy used to say. In a sense, we settled into a pattern of mutual toleration and, with time, even began to accept mediocrity in our relationship as the best we could manage. In my heart, though, this perspective violated my deepest convictions, and I was never totally satisfied that status quo was the way it had to stay. Of course I didn't know that it would take a life-threatening illness before we truly resolved our differences.

One reason we were so anti-divorce was that just before we married, we had come to a position of shared faith. I don't know how Donna ever got me to that particular home Bible study, but I'll never forget the first time I went. I made the mistake of sitting on a squeaky chair. Every time I moved even a little bit, it made a very loud noise. So I sat frozen in place for over thirty minutes while the people prayed. I was trapped. I couldn't wait to get out of there. And I swore I never was going back.

But I did go back, several times, and in the process the Lord just grabbed me. I don't know how else to say it. I began to see a fellowship among the people, a closeness and concern I had never experienced before. As I listened to what they said about salvation, it made sense. I accepted Jesus Christ and invited him into my heart to be my Lord and Savior. Soon after we married, Donna and I were baptized together on a Sunday morning at Central Baptist Church in Norfolk, Virginia.

In December 1977, we rented a U-Haul truck and moved ourselves, our two dogs, and our 18-foot Larson speedboat with 115 horsepower engine to Athens, Tennessee, where I entered a general surgery practice with Dr. Bill Trotter. In some ways, it was like starting a new life. It was refreshing and I enjoyed my work very much. I was doing what I had been training to do for eight long years. And, finally, I was making enough money to pay our bills.

Right away we got involved in a good church, First Baptist Church, which is part of the Southern Baptist Convention. Each week we attended an adult Sunday school class that had a dynamic teacher. One Sunday, Bob Lambert surprised me by asking me to give my testimony, something I had never done before. I fumbled around for a few minutes, telling how I grew up in a religious home, went to church and everything, without ever really coming to know Christ in a personal way. Then I told some of my history through college, how I was searching because I knew there had to be more to life than I had discovered, and how I had finally realized that Jesus was who he said he was.

I would rate that first effort as a C-minus, but evidently it was good enough for Bob, whose motivation became more apparent when he invited me to go to India in 1978 to work with India Youth for Christ on a short-term mission trip. I would be part of the outreach teams, but not practicing medicine.

We broke into seven or eight units on that trip, going out each day to the local villages. We would go into the people's huts, and there on the walls in the semi-darkness were their "gods," grotesque caricatures of what was really the demonic. People there were hungry to know the Lord. Thousands came to Christ during that trip, and for the first time I witnessed healings and exorcisms. Although I wasn't quite sure what to think about all of it, I rejoiced to see the positive response and locked away the rest for future reference.

One thing really did hit me, though: There was obviously an intense need for surgical skills on the mission field. When I returned to the States, I asked about our denomination's short-term medical missions program. In 1979, this program took me to North Yemen, near Saudi Arabia. In 1981, I went to Ghana, West Africa, where I did more than a hundred surgeries in five weeks. Because it was so hot there, I would put a wet towel on the bed before lying down to sleep. I hardly had time to eat a meal, much less speak to any of those patients about faith in Jesus Christ.

This trip was a turning point in our life, however, not because of the work itself, but because I became acquainted with an obstetrician/gynecologist named Andy Norman who, eighteen months later, would deliver the baby who would become our first adopted son.

In 1982, Donna and I decided to go together on a mission trip, this time to Thailand, where I worked as a general practitioner and she as a nurse practitioner in a Cambodian refugee camp. In the back of my mind, I was hoping this experience would nurture our relationship, both maritally and spiritually. But while we did have a great time in Hong Kong, the mission field is hardly the ideal setting to work on a marriage.

We slept in a little hallway with a drawn curtain, but it was so hot and there were so many lizards on the wall and ceiling that it was difficult to get any sleep at all. It was no honeymoon experience, I can assure you! In addition, whether it was the accumulated stress of those three weeks or just our basic personalities jousting again, we had a real blowout on the way home over a little thing like how to fill out the U.S. Customs forms to get back in the country.

Right after we returned, my father died without our being able to talk through some of the things that still nagged me deep inside. I had to try to help Mom through this transition, so I traveled to Georgia every four to six weeks for a long weekend.

Simultaneously, I began thinking about leaving private practice to retrain as a cardiac surgeon. In January 1983 I had just returned from interviewing for a one-year thoracic surgery program in Dallas when we got a call from Andy Norman, who was now practicing in Boone, North Carolina. A young woman in labor who had had no prenatal care walked in off the street and, after delivery, said to Andy, "I don't believe that I can take care of this baby. Would you happen to know someone who would?"

Only a few hours before Jonathan Edward was born, Donna and I had decided to pick up everything and leave our nice house with its four acres, her Master's program and my $100,000 income to enter another residency at one-quarter the pay. When Andy called and asked, "Are you interested in a baby boy?" I had to stop for a minute and ask myself, "Is this really the right time to make a move?"

But because we believed God was opening doors for us, we moved to Dallas in early 1983 and started over, in more ways than one. Suddenly we two had become three—a family—with the result that Donna and I became much closer. Not only that, but my program in Dallas allowed me more time with our infant son than I would ever have had in private practice.

Without a doubt, we were becoming more convinced that the Lord really knew what he was doing. Despite our weaknesses and our strengths, he had been laying a foundation in our life together that would increasingly become more significant and more obvious in the next few years.

That leads me back to where I started this chapter, to the idea of parables and realities. The parable I'm thinking of now, however, is the one that Jesus told at the very end of his famous Sermon on the Mount.

He compared foolish and wise men, and the way they go about building their lives as they build their houses. The

foolish man builds his life upon the sand, for when he hears
Christ's words, he fails to act upon them. When crisis
looms—when the rain comes, the floods rise, and the wind
blows—neither such a house nor such a life can stand. But
the wise person, having heard Christ's words, builds his life
upon them, so that when the storms come, regardless of
how fierce they may be, his house does not fall, because it has
been founded upon a rock.

In reality, this is what preserved our marriage and kept
our home and lives from disintegrating in the storms we
faced in those early years—some of our own creation, and
some beyond our control. Besides the problems already mentioned, we had weathered two malpractice suits while I was
practicing in Tennessee. If there is anything a conscientious
and caring Christian physician doesn't need, it's to be
dragged into court because the results of some procedure
failed to meet somebody's unrealistic expectations. However, I told the Lord that I was ready to accept his will for
the outcomes.

When we were in Dallas, things seemed to level out for
a while, but just on the horizon some clouds were forming
again, specifically the horrendous stress of another residency,
a cardiac surgery program with brutal hours and multiple
responsibilities that would leave me at risk for exposure to a
deadly virus that public-health officials were just beginning to
understand.

△3▷

"Fast Eddie"

*i*n June 1984 we moved to Pittsburgh, Pennsylvania where I had been accepted into a thoracic surgery residency program. My year in Dallas had been spent in a non-accredited fellowship in cardiac, thoracic, and vascular surgery, but it was well worth it and prepared me for Pittsburgh.

That first year at Allegheny was rough, much worse than I remembered my general surgery residency being. I would leave home most mornings between 5:30 and 6:00 and return at 8:00 P.M. If that wasn't crazy enough, when I was on call, I stayed right through and worked all night at the hospital, followed by another full shift before I got home again. You hardly have time or energy to wonder why you're doing this (or why you're allowing somebody else to do it to you!). You just beat yourself, like the long line of surgeons before you—trying to prove something. Just *what* is anybody's guess.

Since you've probably never been inside the doors of an operating room, let me give you a quick glimpse behind the scenes. As you look over my shoulder, you'll easily see how a surgeon might get exposed to HIV (or, more commonly, to hepatitis B), especially if he or she works very fast. And *I* was fast enough to earn the nickname "Fast Eddie" when I was a general surgical resident in Norfolk. Maybe I was too fast for my own good, especially on that unknown day in the spring of 1985.

It is now 7:30 A.M., and I've already made rounds on yesterday's patients. I've taken out some chest tubes and some balloons (inserted into the large artery in the chest from the groin artery to temporarily assist while the heart itself recovers from the shock of surgery), and I've written some patient transfer orders.

Now I head for the operating room, where I take another look at the films (coronary angiograms or X-rays), scrub, put on my gloves, and prepare the already anesthetized patient for surgery. (Don't be surprised—residents open and close most of the cases in our program.) I help insert a large intravenous line, down through the patient's neck and into the heart area. Then I drape out the chest and legs, since we usually use the greater saphenous vein from the thigh for several of the bypass grafts.

Next I make an incision down the center of the sternum (breastbone), using a scalpel until I actually hit the bone. The next cut is made with a small power-driven saw, taking care to stay in the middle. Don't worry, the patient doesn't feel a thing. Actually, it's much easier than it looks, especially since this is the first time his chest has been opened. I hook the tip of the saw under the xiphoid (the back of the sternum) and *Zip! Zip!* I'm already done. Maybe you've already seen enough, but we're just getting started. Aren't you amazed how bloodless this whole thing has been so far? I'll just stop that little bit of bleeding on the edges of the sternum with some bone wax.

Now it's time to put in a chest spreader, to keep the cavity open while we work on the heart. I slowly crank open the retractor, being very careful not to break the ribs, and not to tear the innominate vein that crosses the chest at the top of the incision.

I carefully slit the pericardium and suspend it with stitches to the retractor or edge of the incision. Next I put "purse string" sutures in a circle on the aorta, the big artery that comes out of the heart, and on the appendage of the atrium where the blood returns to the heart. I leave the ends long, sliding a piece of rubber over the atrium's appendage, to be tightened down around the tubing when we go on bypass. A large tube is then placed in the right atrium after the patient's blood is thinned with heparin. Finally, I insert a small piece of plastic tubing into the aorta, secure it, and connect both cannulas to tubing from the heart/lung machine.

Everything's ready now. The patient is connected, above and below the heart, to the machine that will sustain his life while we stop his heart long enough to make repairs. I have the attending surgeon called. So far, as you see, he hasn't even been in the room.

He walks in, looks everything over very carefully, and finally says, "Okay, Dr. Rozar, it's your turn." Just what I've been waiting to hear! "Let's go," I say to the well-trained team as everybody swings into action. The heart/lung machine begins its work of pumping blood through the patient's system. The large artery arising out of the heart is clamped to isolate the heart so it can be emptied. But the heart keeps beating until it is iced down and a special drug called cardioplegia, which stops and protects it, is infused into the heart.

The heart is still now, and I look for the vessels on the heart (often hard to find because of fatty tissue) and mark them with a small incision. Next I measure to see how long a vein is needed, cut off the right length, and connect the distal end to the coronary artery below the blockage, thus "bypassing" it. After I've done this in two different areas, the third and final bypass today is done using the left internal mammary artery. The free end is connected to a vessel of the heart where increased circulation is needed. (This internal mammary artery was taken down after the chest was opened and before car- diopulmonary bypass commenced.)

Once we have finished working on the heart and every- thing checks out, we remove the large clamp on the aorta so that the heart has blood coursing through it again. The ends of the veins are then sewn to the aorta and flow is established in the "bypasses." (The origin of the mammary artery is already attached by God to the artery of the arm.) Cardiopulmonary bypass is terminated after the patient is warmed up and all sites look good. The attending surgeon leaves for another case. (Closing the chest, like opening, is also usually the job of a resident.). It is not a glorious job, but it is an important part of the procedure. Total time, skin to skin, is 3 hours, 20 minutes, longer than acceptable to me, but faster than most.

I hope I haven't grossed you out completely by that very brief and far too simplistic explanation of what I used to do—a typical episode in the workday of a surgical resident. Since I was usually involved with at least two heart surgeries a day, plus rounds before and after, the hours flew past, even if the cases were first-time procedures and everything went well.

"Redos" (what we call subsequent chest openings in people who have had heart surgery before) were another story altogether. Stuff can end up flying all over the place and whoever is doing the cutting can end up covered with blood. This isn't a problem in terms of the patient because there is plenty of blood available for transfusion as needed. But you would be appalled (and I am now as I think back) how bloody things sometimes get in there.

The second time around, the heart is usually right up against the breastbone, and we have to use a different saw (a sidebiting saw) without a guard on its blade. The surgeon must be very careful, holding the saw with one hand and guiding it with the other, as cuts are made first through the outer table (of the sternum) and then through the inner table. This is delicate business with little room for error. If you get into the right ventricle of the heart by cutting too deeply, everybody in the room, especially the patient, has a very big problem.

It is not so much the blood that may splatter on you while you work that risks the transmission of diseases like HIV or hepatitis B. More likely, one way or another you'll end up sticking yourself with "sharps": needles or maybe a scalpel. Because you use magnification (magnifying lenses attached to the front of what look like normal eyeglasses) to be certain the delicate sutures are placed correctly, you have a tunnel view and a small field to look at as you work. No matter how careful you are, you can get stuck, or stick somebody else, as you race against the clock. If you have to look up to hand something to an attendant or receive something yourself, you might as well start over. The whole situation is intense: The heart is stopped, and the length of time it is stopped is important. You know if something goes wrong, you're going to need every extra second. So I've stuck people that way, and I've been stuck myself, many times, either with a very small needle or even with the big ones used to close the chest.

I hate to think how often I stuck myself while closing a case (I participated in over 250 heart cases during my residency alone). It was just too easy to puncture my own hand with the sternal wire needle I was trying to push through the bone or even around it, while lifting the breastbone underneath with the other hand. For reasons that are obvious, I would rather stick my own hand or finger than the patient's heart.

Sometimes I had to work blind, by feel. If I got stuck, I didn't even think about it—just changed a glove, or maybe not, but kept going, whatever happened. I might see blood in my glove after I finished and have no idea how or when it got there. Even if I noticed it while still working, I would ignore it for the sake of speed.

Anyone who sews by hand can identify with this. What happens when you're doing a stiff seam with one hand inside, while the other pushes the needle through? Well, multiply that by a factor of a thousand to allow for the pressure of human flesh versus denim, and you can easily see why surgeons stick themselves so often—and why they're so concerned about doing invasive and sometimes blind procedures on HIV-positive patients.

But that is still not the whole story of a day in the life of Ed Rozar, resident physician. Maybe I did get infected in the operating room, but I did a lot more than open and close cases for attending surgeons or do skin-to-skin procedures. What happened in the controlled environment of the operating room was a piece of cake compared to what I might encounter in the intensive care unit after hours. I often stood between a recovering patient's emergency and his or her sudden death.

A significant percentage of heart patients have complications, especially soon after their surgery. These problems can be minor or major, depending on the patient and the type of surgery performed. If a patient dropped his blood pressure or maybe developed a clot around the heart after surgery, I would have to cut him open right there, take the stitches out, and open the chest to expose the heart. That meant cutting wires and spreading the chest by hand—lots of opportunity for puncture wounds from metal and bone. Or if a patient went baseline (no heartbeat), I couldn't push on the chest to restart the heart because the sternum had just been wired and was now two bones instead of one. So I had to open the chest quickly and compress the heart by hand.

Once I had two patients in crisis, lying side by side with their chests open. Fortunately, I have long arms, and they were both within my reach. I can't recall compressing a heart with each hand, but when I got one patient back, the other one arrested and I just turned and went to the other bed. Those were the wildest few minutes I ever had. Fortunately, both patients survived. During times like these it would have been easy enough to puncture a glove, or get scratched or stuck in that frenzy of activity. What was I supposed to do then? Stop and change gloves? Give a lecture on "universal precautions"?

Sometimes as a resident I would be called to the emergency department. And there is no doubt in my mind that I took care of many patients who, when they were later admitted, were officially listed as someone else's. Consequently, any "look back" studies (examining the records of all patients in that institution associated with my name as a physician) might still never solve the question that seems more important to others than it is to me: Who was the patient who gave me HIV?

I'm not bitter about this, and the only reason I would want to know now is that I might be able to let that person know about his or her HIV status. Most likely, however, whoever it was is either very sick or already dead, probably the latter.

Of course, I now had acquired a deadly disease without my knowledge. I was feeling well enough that spring—chalking up any fatigue to the horrendous pace of the program, which was about to let up a little. My final year there, starting in July, would consist of a more varied schedule. I was to be on an elective rotation in July. Looking back, it would also be a time to recover from the acute, debilitating illness I had in May 1985.

Beyond that, we became the proud adoptive parents of another son in April. One day our pastor's wife called Donna and said, "A pastor-friend of ours has a woman in his church who is pregnant but wants to give up the child. Do you know anybody who'd be interested in a baby?"

"Well, yes. Us!" Donna replied, without even consulting me. Not that I would have argued against it. David was born on April 12, and we picked him up on April 15. Again, this brought us closer. Now we had two sons to love, and that, probably more than anything else, put our unresolved differences on hold.

Just two weeks after we welcomed David into our home, I traveled to New Orleans to attend a conference of the American Association of Thoracic Surgeons. On May 1, 1985, I was at a fine restaurant having dinner with my department chairman and several other attending surgeons from Allegheny when suddenly I started having a strange feeling in my neck—a cross between irritation and pain. I rubbed it, but it didn't go away. And I felt hot.

I looked around the table to see if anybody else was sick, thinking maybe it was the food. But no one else seemed to be affected. I managed to finish dinner, made it back to my room, took some aspirin, and went to bed. By the next morning, I felt bad enough to miss the meeting, though I did recover enough by dinnertime to go out with a fellow resident and his wife.

That was my last good meal for quite a while. Overnight I was sick again and feeling totally washed out. By the time I got on the plane to go home Thursday, I was miserable. That flight was the most difficult I ever hope to have, complete with fever, nausea, aches, and assorted pains. I just lay back and tried to survive it. I was one sick puppy, that's for sure.

I was supposed to work the next morning, but that was impossible. I was just too sick. Fortunately, that weekend I was not on call, so I stayed in bed the whole time. By Monday, when I showed up on schedule in the operating room, I still wasn't feeling much better. In fact, for the first time in my entire medical career, I had to be excused from the operating room to go out and vomit. When it happened again later that same week, they sent me home until I could get over whatever was wrong with me.

The next couple of weeks are still fuzzy in my mind. I remember seeing a physician at an attending surgeon's request, but I also remember that Donna had to drive me to the hospital for the lab tests because I was too weak to drive.

After $600 worth of tests, my doctor concluded I had a mononucleosis type of viral illness. The symptoms were classic of an acute HIV infection: fatigue, aches and pains, nausea, no appetite. In fact, I couldn't eat anything except Popsicles for several weeks. Even ice cream, which I had always loved, had become distasteful. That was strange, I thought, but that was about as far as I went with it. The whole thing was bizarre.

Nobody ever suggested doing an HIV screen. Apparently nobody even thought about it, maybe because as far as anyone knew, AIDS was a disease afflicting certain patient populations, and there was no chance a health-care worker could get it from a patient. (That was the information put out at the time and, in fact, continued for several more years.) Remember, it wasn't until April or May of 1985 that the blood banks started routinely screening for HIV on "banked blood," though not patients.

I got little sympathy from my colleagues, either attending surgeons or fellow residents. When you're a resident, the work is pretty cruel and grueling—almost like slave labor. I got all sorts of flack for missing work, but ignored most of it. They really expected me to just dive back into the routine. I had never hidden from work before, but now it was necessary to slow down a little so that I could recover from this "unknown" illness.

The program was doing a total of eight hearts a day, sometimes more. Since there were only two junior thoracic residents, one senior and one fellow, every warm body was needed to assist, especially since the attending surgeons counted on us to get the cases going. Then they might have one of us "do" the procedure if we were qualified and technically ready. They were really doing us a favor by letting us do so much, but with increased participation comes increased responsibility. Some attending surgeons seem to think they're doing residents a favor just by letting them be there, but at our program everything was okay as long as you put forth the effort. I suppose there was the feeling that we did owe them something, but that's true of most training programs.

One of the attending surgeons actually tried to get my week's vacation revoked because I had been out with this illness. That maneuver failed, and I took my vacation, which I spent recovering. When I finally returned to work early in June, I discovered I was now on call every other night for three weeks. I had no choice but to grit my teeth and tough it out, though I knew it would be a grueling month. Here I was just starting to feel better, even starting to eat again—I had lost twenty pounds during the acute phase of the illness.

Because I was nearly always totally exhausted by the time I had survived another thirty-six-hour stint, I would go home, crawl in a hole, and wish I could die. I was in a survival mode and felt like a zombie sometimes, but I had to be really careful because I still had to make life-and-death decisions every day. I am sure that it was supernatural strength that sustained me. "The LORD is my strength and my shield; my heart trusts in Him, and I am helped . . ." (Ps. 28:7).

One of the things that kept me going, I guess, was that I knew it would only last a month. The new "slaves" would be arriving July 1, and I wouldn't be the clinical chief anymore. I could do an elective, selecting cases to meet my board requirements, which meant I would have a lighter schedule for July.

During July, I did get a little more rest, and by August I had basically recovered. After that, I tried to ignore that episode of sickness, maybe because I was still pretty busy. I had no other symptoms to speak of, but I was never able to regain those twenty pounds, although I had returned to a regular diet, including ice cream. I wondered about that weight loss from time to time, especially when somebody would mention I looked thin. I would just reply, "Yeah, I used to weigh 170." I was down to 150, and my biggest problem seemed to be how to buy a new wardrobe on a resident's salary, with three other mouths to feed.

Obviously, I never really forgot that illness in 1985, especially the dramatic weight loss and my inability to regain weight. Every time I looked in the mirror after a shower, I was reminded. But it never crossed my mind to seek another medical opinion. I was feeling well enough again, and I had a lot more important things to worry about. What career direction would be best for me and my growing family once my residency was finished? Would I be able to pass my board-certification exams, written and then oral?

4

King of the Hill

*i*magine holding a little premature baby, not much bigger than two hands. This tiny newborn has a hole, about the diameter of a pencil, between the two chambers of his heart (a VSD), which itself is about the size of a small orange. If somebody doesn't fix that defect, this child has little chance of seeing his first birthday. If the baby survives infancy, every normal childhood physical activity will be a supreme effort, perhaps even a threat to his life.

That's what keeps people like Dr. Robert (Gus) Gustafson operating. During a rotation from November 1985 to February 1986, I became acquainted with Gus, who was professor of pediatric thoracic surgery at West Virginia University School of Medicine in Morgantown. I enjoyed the work so much, especially working with Gus, that I seriously considered doing a fellowship (another one-year residency) in pediatric heart surgery.

A couple of things stopped me. For one thing, I didn't relish the idea of playing the resident game anymore. For another, the work was so delicate and the patients so fragile

41

that unless you have at least one expert associate, a pediatric cardiac surgeon might as well move into the hospital. Donna wasn't too keen on that idea, and I realized, too, that I didn't want my sons growing up without me.

About the biggest problem I encountered during that rotation was finding enough space for Donna and the boys to visit me on weekends. I had been provided the usual accommodations—one room. When I mentioned I had a wife and two kids and needed more space, at first they said I would have to pay for it. But on a resident's salary, we were just making ends meet. Dr. Gordon Murray, who was chief of thoracic surgery at the time, intervened and found me a small three-bedroom apartment in the faculty housing dorm. The family would come down from Pittsburgh on a Thursday and stay until Sunday. I never had time to be lonely when they weren't there, because of the immense amount of reading I had to do to get up to speed with this fascinating specialty.

Although I finally decided against another fellowship, Gus was instrumental in getting me a position as assistant professor of surgery at West Virginia University School of Medicine. So we ended up working together anyway—not too bad for a guy without the kind of credentials normally expected. I think Gus and Dr. Murray wanted me on board mainly for my clinical skills.

We moved to Morgantown in the summer of 1986. Donna wasn't exactly excited about going there, and the salary was maybe 60 percent of what I might have made elsewhere. But we reminded each other that making a lot of money was never a big deal for me anyway. One thing I will say for it, though, the position came with some good benefits, including a pension plan that put away each year an equivalent of 20 percent of my salary.

I really liked working with the residents and medical students. On a typical day we would do one or two heart surgeries, mostly bypasses, but we also did valve replacements and some lung surgery. I think I did ninety-five hearts my first year there, which was quite a few, considering that the next closest surgeon's total was seventy-five. So I made some money for the university—they knew it and so did I—and as a result I got a little bonus.

The boys were growing up so fast, and I enjoyed the time I had with them. It was fascinating to see these two together. The love they gave each other spilled over into our whole family. But my colleagues had subtle ways of letting me know that even when not on call, for instance on a weekend, I was still supposed to make rounds if I was in town.

"Aren't you coming by?" they would ask.

"I'm off," I would reply. "I wasn't planning to come back until Monday."

"Why not?"

I regret how often I gave in to the pressure to make Sunday-morning rounds on patients and as a result miss church, but I still had enough time off to satisfy us. We managed that winter to do something we had wanted to do for a long time; we learned to snow ski, at Canaan Valley, West Virginia—a great place for kids.

We also enjoyed the water, and by our second summer in West Virginia had fallen in love with sailing. One weekend in August, we all spent three nights on a sailboat with another young couple. We rented a thirty-five-foot sailboat near Annapolis and sailed the Chesapeake Bay, though we almost returned with one less Rozar. Jonathan and David were playing tug-of-war with a rope, Jonathan in the galley and David on deck. Suddenly, Jonathan let go and David went flying. Fortunately for us, I was sitting there beside him, watching them play. I reached out by instinct and snagged him just before he would have flipped overboard.

We returned home with the same number of kids after that trip, but it wasn't long before our "quiver" filled up all at once. For some time we had been trying to adopt again, through a local agency. We learned in the process that if we wanted to get a young child, the only way would be to take either one with special needs or a sibling group. We had requested siblings, if possible.

At one point three girls had been available for adoption, but we didn't get them. We learned later that we were considered "too intelligent" and our kids "too motivated" for these three girls to fit into our family. The social workers felt that they probably wouldn't be able to "adjust." Another set of parents got the girls, and then wound up giving them back. I don't know what happened to them, but such is the world of adoption procedures, as anybody knows who's been through it.

We really didn't know what the Lord had in mind during this time of disappointment. It was disheartening to Donna, and I must confess I was hurt by the agency's rationale. But then, out of the blue, we got another call. Would we drive down to Beckley, West Virginia, about three hours south? A social worker there had three children she wanted us to meet.

I'll never forget that day. Before I tell you what the kids were like when we took them in, I assure you that today they are all doing fine, and we're very proud of the progress they have made. Our family has grown together by God's grace and all the kids love each other. It is amazing how they get along, considering their various backgrounds and genetic makeup. Jonathan Edward continues to be the leader and having four siblings has helped him mature. David is our video and computer kid who loves all the interaction with so many kids. Victoria has developed into a beautiful girl and has taken on the "mother hen" role when she relates to the three younger children. Jonathan Wayne continues to be very active. He is our "jock" but a very precious boy. Christina has also developed into a beautiful young girl. I suppose she will always be our "baby."

On arriving in Beckley, we checked into a motel. Soon the social workers came with the three kids. It was quite an experience. Christina, sixteen months old, sat quietly on the bed. She had no expression on her face and did not respond to affection. Jonathan Wayne (he was already named before he became a Rozar), who was almost three, was simply hyper—running back and forth from room to room. Four-year-old Victoria just wanted to sit and watch TV. She didn't yet know her colors or the names of animals.

Christina, who had been in a foster home different from the one Jonathan Wayne and Victoria were in, brought a letter with her describing a very regimented schedule—at 9 o'clock you have to do this; at 10 this, and so on, almost as if life in that home had been organized entirely around her needs. She was still on the bottle, but the worst thing was that somehow her little stuffed puppy dog had been left behind. She screamed bloody murder for several hours that night—the kids stayed with us overnight at the motel—and we didn't know why.

That wasn't the biggest surprise, by a long shot. The next day—Sunday—the social worker showed up in the morning with all their toys and clothes. Overnight, our family of four had mushroomed to seven, without our even having a chance to go home and think it over! The local head of the private adoption agency was livid. Evidently, procedures had been bent. "You're not supposed to bring those children home— they never do that," she said. "You're not supposed to have those children now."

I've concluded that it would have been light-years easier to have had triplets, and I'm not sure how anybody survives that! The adjustment required of everybody during the next few months defies description. For some reason, Jonathan Wayne became violent, destroying things like antique furniture. It seemed he couldn't stop until whatever it was he was attacking was broken.

I couldn't even get near Christina for six months. She would just scream, or alternate between screaming and sitting on the bed with no expression. It was really bizarre, and it took eight months—maybe a year—before we could become close.

Victoria still just wanted to sit and watch TV.

On top of all that, Jonathan Edward and David had to adjust, too. David rebelled, regressed, and lost a lot of ground when the other three kids arrived. Jonathan Edward was still too young to have his own bedroom, so for a while we had three boys in the same room, using a set of bunks and a youth bed.

Perhaps the biggest conflict for the first two boys in our family was about ownership. I don't know how often we heard, "That was mine before you came," whether in relation to toys, games, or even the bedroom itself.

Of all the shocks to our family stability, however, the most disturbing came about eight months after the last three kids moved in with us, a time when our lives had finally hit some kind of normalcy. Our lives were suddenly thrown into turmoil when someone filed a complaint of child abuse. One day in the spring of 1988, we got called down to the child protection agency (CPA), where one bitter woman presented us with a list of complaints. The most serious one was the charge by an unidentified witness (the accused in such cases have no right to know their accuser) that David had been seen with bruises on his bottom. You would have thought we were in Hitler's office, being branded as high criminals. This dictator had a long list of demands, including that we put the children in school—a nonreligious school (we were home-schooling). The younger ones must attend day care, and we were not to use any form of corporal punishment on the children.

The woman at CPA had us over a barrel, and she knew it. The last three kids hadn't yet been legally adopted. And now there was this formal complaint, and we were being investigated. Without doubt, it was her goal to take those kids away from us.

Nonetheless, I must admit I was less than cordial in my response. "You can't do that," I replied, waving the paper in her face. "You're infringing on my rights. This is America. I won't agree to this. It's garbage! You can try, but we'll fight you all the way."

Donna kept telling me to cool it, but I wasn't listening. "No way," I said. "This is wrong. We have to stand up for our rights."

I let it be known that if somebody tried to take away the kids, I would sue. "We'll be glad to go through this investigation," I said. "I'm going to get a lawyer, too."

It was a very hostile confrontation—one of the most difficult spots I've ever been in. This woman was trying to destroy us, especially what we stood for. To me, it was as simple as that.

To be fair, it's possible David did have a few mild bruises on his bottom. He had been having a tough time for months, rebelling when the others came. But, in our own defense, he was born with what are known as "Mongolian spots," bluish splotches on his buttocks, which might easily be taken for bruises by someone who had never seen them before (we found out later who it was).

I told that CPA woman about David's spots and that they were well documented by his pediatrician. "So this is all libel and slander," I shouted. "There's not a word of truth to it. We don't abuse our children; we love them." When I finished, that woman's face was about the same color as the spots in question.

At a cost of several thousand dollars, we retained a Christian lawyer, who thought we might have to take it to the Rutherford Institute and focus on the religious-freedom aspects of the case. We had many people praying, too, because this kind of thing is not just a personal attack, it is spiritual warfare.

Talk about being paranoid, we knew the CPA had the power to come get the children, no matter what I said. So we were concerned about not spanking the children, because someone might hear them carrying on and report us again. But we sometimes did have to spank Jonathan Wayne because, even after all that time, he was still a wild colt in need of a corral. Of course, I love him to death, and we've had some great times together, snowmobiling at the farm and things like that. It took us a while to get there, however.

Sometime later—and I'm glad I wasn't home—the CPA worker showed up at the house. Donna said she was like a totally different person. She just sat on the floor and played games with the kids and then left. Although that was the last we saw of her, it was a very tough period, especially after everything we had gone through to take these children into our home. To feel like criminals, afraid to live the way we knew was right, was a test—another very strong test of our foundations.

But again, we emerged intact. The storm just made us stronger. A week before Thanksgiving of 1988, the judge, who had perhaps heard we were about to move to Wisconsin, where I had accepted a position at the Marshfield Clinic, scheduled us to appear before him.

What a scene that was! Here we were in a typical small-town West Virginia courthouse, standing before a judge who had five kids of his own, for a hearing that would decide the fate of three children we had come to love deeply. The kids were crawling under the table, and the judge was laughing. David sat on the judge's knee while he asked us a few questions. Interestingly enough, he never asked us about the allegations of child abuse. One of our favorite photos has all of us crowded around that judge in that little courtroom, with everybody smiling and very happy, including him. Before we left, we finalized everything, and Jonathan Wayne, Victoria, and Christina were officially Rozars—ours forever. The charges of child abuse were dropped and the case was closed. Thank you, Lord.

That one word, *ours,* is the key to that whole transition. When we moved to Marshfield, a friendly dairy town of 18,000 set among central Wisconsin's gently rolling glacial hills, everything became *ours.* We moved into *our* new house together, a beautiful two-story, four-bedroom brick house with blue-gray siding, big enough for everybody to have his or her own space. The full basement was great for *our* home-schooling. The wooded lot with its big backyard meant there was room for a gym and a sandbox and a clubhouse and a swing set for *our* kids to share with *our* neighbors. This family-oriented kind of community—where people are less impressed that you are a cardiac surgeon than whether you've been to your kid's Little League game—was *our* kind of town—home. Without a doubt, we were on top of the world.

In terms of my work, I was now making more money than I ever thought I would, but that just meant we would have more to give away. I was busy, too. Despite its rural location, the Marshfield Clinic is one of the largest and finest heart-surgery centers in the country. As I recall, I did four hearts the first week, plus an emergency consult my very first day. In the first five months I probably did forty to fifty heart cases, but I was also doing pulmonary consults and some lung surgery.

In spite of that, I still had time to work on a paper about a special incision I had developed to save the chest wall muscle in thoracic procedures. I had done maybe fifteen cases that way, but it wasn't quite enough to publish.

I was on call every night during the week, but lived only several minutes from the hospital. On weekends, if I wasn't on call, I didn't have to worry about the patients at all. Because there were three other cardiac surgeons who shared call, you were free from Friday afternoon until Monday morning on the weekends that you were off. This freedom was a greater benefit than a large salary.

Besides having three out of four weekends off, there were other benefits. Life, disability, medical, and dental insurance—the works—was part of the employment contract. This factor was to be far more providential than I ever could have guessed when I took the position.

During the winter, we went skiing, trying to teach the two youngest boys to ski. We went to Powderhorn, in Michigan's Upper Peninsula, and had a lot of fun. The kids learned to ice skate, too. And we went sledding. Since I was on call only about one weekend a month, I had a lot more time with the family.

Physically, I was fatigued and had more back trouble than ever. So, in January 1989, I had a complete employment physical by a physician who later felt bad that he didn't see the HIV. But all my lab work was normal, except for a slightly elevated lymphocyte count. Everything else was okay. I attributed my weariness to the move and the recent legal hassles, but mostly to the fact that surgery is always so tiring that you don't think anything about it, unless you're so totally wiped out you can't move. Since I was now doing every procedure myself, skin to skin, a little fatigue was nothing to worry about.

If anything *was* clear, it was that God had abundantly provided for us and had chosen to bless us more than we could have imagined. Everything was as if I had written out, "This is what I want to do, Lord. Can you fix it for me?" He did it—almost like the happy ending to *The Ed Rozar Family Fairy Tale*.

But one day in April 1989, when I was between an open-heart case and a lung case, our fairy tale got fractured by fourteen words said to me over the phone. A few weeks earlier I had decided to change a whole-life insurance policy that was costing about three hundred dollars a month into a term policy through the American College of Surgeons (ACS). Besides all the forms to fill out, a perfunctory blood test was required. I had sent it in without giving it a second thought.

Then came the phone call. The ACS representative asked, first, if I had applied for insurance. "Yes," I replied, wondering only vaguely what the problem might be.

"I don't know how to tell you this," he hesitated, "but your HIV test was positive."

Stunned, I hung up the phone, my normal decisiveness suddenly overwhelmed by a multitude of questions, like a black cloud in the middle of a sunny day. *How can this be true? I'm healthy as a horse. This can't be happening. There must be some mistake! I am in a no-risk group.*

Stifling the emotional eruption for a moment, my scientific mind needed facts and some solid, informed advice. Believe it or not, what came to my mind first wasn't myself, my wife, or my kids. It was: *Should I operate on my next patient?*

Quickly I called Dr. Doug Lee, an infectious-disease specialist. After we talked it all over, the best route seemed to be to submit two more tests, anonymously, one to the local lab and one to a lab in Minnesota. Doug was confident it was just a false positive. After all, how could it be true? I didn't fit the HIV profile. At this point, there was no reason to cancel any surgeries, certainly not until the lab results were back.

Next I called Donna, who was downstairs with the kids when the phone rang. "A pathologist from Dallas called today to tell me my HIV screen was positive," I told her.

"Oh," she replied. "Oh—you're kidding me!" It took a moment to register.

"No," I responded, as calmly as I could manage, looking out at the gray early spring sky and wishing I knew more answers myself. "I've talked the whole thing over with Dr. Doug Lee. We're sending out another sample. Maybe it's just a false positive."

I hung up, and sat at my desk, trying to collect my thoughts: *Everything is down the drain, all washed up. My career is over, maybe my life is over.* I didn't know much about AIDS yet, but I knew it spelled death. *What about the kids? What about the house? What will we do if I can't operate?* My mind was wheeling a million miles an hour. In a matter of minutes, I had tumbled from the top of the hill—in charge, in control—to the bottom. Despite Doug's reassurance, I had an intuition that in the near future I would become more a patient than a physician.

In those quiet moments, I reached for the one thing I knew I could trust, my Bible: the Word of God. I kept it in the office to read while waiting for patients to stabilize. My mind was confused enough that I can't recall what I read. But when I put it down, I had a sense that God was there, and because of that, I didn't need to be afraid.

There had to be some trembling. My epinephrine level and heart rate were probably sky-high. As a surgeon, I lived with crisis all the time, but this was my crisis, which certainly put it in a different light. But that day, at least, there were no tears. I had to get back to work. A patient was waiting, the staff was standing by. If I was going to become a patient myself, so be it. For the next couple of hours, however, this surgeon would have to put his skills on automatic pilot. I would have to depend on an inner peace "that passes all understanding" to keep my hands steady and my mind focused on the task I had trained so long and hard to do.

5

Life on Hold

*a*lmost immediately, the local lab report, using the ELISA test (the initial test for HIV antibodies), confirmed the ACS report. From then on, I had no doubt I would have to give up surgery. But somehow we held on to what hope we had through the intervening weekend, awaiting the definitive Western Blot test results that should be back by Monday. I was on call both weekend nights and making rounds on thirty to forty patients twice a day, so the time flew by. But I'll always remember it as the longest weekend of my life.

Donna and I were going through the motions of living, working, and doing things with the kids. Our life was on hold, as if we were in a dream or a trance. You wake up in the morning, walk into the bathroom, look at yourself in the mirror, and wonder if it can possibly be real. And you ask yourself, a thousand times a day, *How can it be real?* You might even whisper, "God, I'm glad it's not real."

Reality hit, full force, that Monday, when Doug brought the results to my office. I could see it in his face before he said the words. And no doubt he could see what I was feel-

53

ing before either of us spoke. "The Western Blot is positive, too," he said quietly. "I'm sorry."

Now what? I wondered. I could hear Doug continue talking, though my mind and emotions were now threatening to disconnect.

"We'll have to get some others involved," he said. When I nodded, he added, "I'll talk it over confidentially with Reed Hall (the clinic's general counsel). He'll need to call around to see what's happened elsewhere, but he won't find anything. There's not yet been even one report of reverse transmission from a health-care worker to a patient. I don't see why you can't keep operating until we get a ruling."

At that point I wasn't in any mood for an argument, but my thought was: *Even if it's one chance in a million, or one in ten million, that's one too many.* For that one person it's a hundred percent, as it was for me.

Only a few days later, I laid down my surgeon's knife for the final time. It was as much a legal and ethical question as anything else. I knew it was both the prudent and the right thing to do, whether or not a nationwide search had turned up a precedent. I closed that last case with a sigh of regret that I hadn't achieved my potential. *What a shame,* I thought. *What a waste.* It wasn't as if I was ending my career at the normal retirement age. *Here I am, forty years old. They just spent all that money to recruit and move me here. I won't even be able to pay them back for that.* Funny what mixed thoughts go through your mind at such a time.

It was a lung case, as I recall, not that difficult by comparison to some others I had done, but each case had been important to me in a special way. Some had been emergency situations where the patient would have died if I had not made the right split-second decisions. Yet even the most "minor" procedure challenged my know-how. Each case was not just a name on a chart, but a person, and I had always enjoyed talking to my patients and their families. Saving lives and helping more people get better is why I had gone through that grueling retraining experience.

Now I was sad and frustrated, wondering whether it had been worth it. "You're useless now," I told myself. "Finished!" More than anything, I had a feeling of emptiness, futility. Instead of contemplating a new chapter in my life, I found that somebody had ripped out the rest of the pages. In an emotional sense, I had been violated and felt helpless. I had gone from being a capable and respected heart surgeon to nothingness. Even my M.D. had no meaning anymore.

In the midst of my discouragement, two men were like shining lights. Reed Hall, the clinic's counsel, kept saying, "Don't worry, Ed. We'll find something for you. And don't worry about insurance. All of the health, life, and disability insurance will be kept in place. You need it now more than ever. If the disability is not approved for a year, we'll pay your salary. You have more important things to think about."

My other pillar of support was Dr. Doug Lee, who right from the start was as positive as possible, despite mounting lab evidence that my immune system had been compromised for some time. My blood count showed T4-cells (white blood cells processed through the thymus gland) at 230 (normal is 1,000), with a T4-T8 ratio of 0.15 (normal is 1.0). I'll have more to say in the next chapter about how HIV works, but the loud and clear message for me was: Get help, as soon as possible! I knew my risk of opportunistic infection was great. The main help available at that point was a relatively new drug called AZT, which we decided to start as soon as possible: April 28, 1989, at 11:00 A.M.

As Doug and I traced my history, it became increasingly clear that my initial HIV infection had occurred during my residency at Allegheny General Hospital. Working forward from that period, he computed something else, that my life expectancy was now only about three years—1992! It was time for him to make a house call.

I was in and out of the den during Doug's visit to our home, since I still had patients in different stages of recovery and every few minutes I would be paged to call the hospital.

Once, Donna was in tears when I came back. Later she told me that Doug had been very candid. "Enjoy the summer," he said, "because I can't promise you'll have another one." She could hardly believe her ears. On the other hand, when somebody levels with you like that, it's highly unlikely you have misunderstood what's been said. I guess it was Doug's way of saying, "This is serious. You better get your house in order, just in case."

On the other hand, he tried to paint as bright a picture as possible of the way things might go with AZT, which had shown some promise of delaying the onset of AIDS in asymptomatic patients. "You can improve," he told me. "You're going to feel better than you have in a long time. I hope your immune system will stabilize. You're probably not going to have any side effects."

Besides *my* health, Doug was also very concerned about Donna's HIV status. Considering the fact that we had been enjoying intimate sex the whole time I had been infected, he wanted to ensure at least three things: Donna should get tested as soon as possible; she should have her own internist monitor her situation; and we should be very "careful" from now on in terms of sexual intimacy.

I think if there was anything that lit Donna's fuse, it was this. But I should let her say it in her own words:

> That bothered me the most, that this thing had even invaded our bedroom. That made me really angry. I could cope with all the other things, but to think that this unseen invader had now stolen something that was so good. How can it do that? Here was such a positive part of our marriage and there had never been any fear, there had never been any problem, and suddenly HIV comes and just ruins it all. I just felt it wasn't fair.

With all the stuff being written in the popular press, it was hard to figure why she was still HIV-negative when I had been infected since 1985. Maybe it was the providence of God. If it was, did we dare test providence further by continuing as before—or even by continuing with the use of a condom, with its reported annual failure rate of at least 15 percent?

This problem is far more complicated than it might seem on the surface. I tell you about it not because I want to—we're really quite private people—but because some can't understand why, with all the latex barriers available today, anybody could be dumb enough to risk infection with a deadly disease for a few moments of pleasure.

Donna and I are spontaneous people, so beyond the fact that sex with condoms is less enjoyable, it is also far less impromptu. Within a marriage where two people are firmly committed to each other, it is very difficult to remove this aspect without diminishing the broader mutual meaning that the sexual act seems intended to have. It's near impossible, believe me, to relax and enjoy sex—even if you're using all the protections modern science has to offer—when in the back of your mind is the word: *transmission, transmission, transmission.*

Perhaps this has not been such an issue for us as it might be for others, since for a while I was so sick I didn't have the energy or interest required for sexual performance. But I certainly had a need that sex seems designed by God to help fulfill—a need for intimacy. I was lonely, often quite discouraged. In a very real sense, I was dealing with the death of my dreams. And, as Rebekah comforted Isaac after his mother's death, I needed a similar kind of comfort from my wife.

On the other hand, I think we men often overlook the importance this part of marriage also has to our wives. They need that closeness, too, perhaps even more than we do, so it's no wonder Donna was so offended when this illness suddenly threatened me, and therefore her, in many ways.

Early on, we gently argued about "safe sex." This may not seem as humorous to you as it is to us, looking back, but one night she protested: "It's not going to kill me," and I replied, "Oh, yes, it will," feeling like a leper or worse. Total abstinence would have been the simplest solution, of course, and perhaps the most prudent for the sake of the children. But I think the best long-range solution is to find creative new routes to intimacy and closeness, as some physically disabled people have done.

For a long time after I got the Western Blot report, I felt a bit paranoid, and not just in terms of Donna. When I needed some dental work, I wasn't sure what to do. But Doug Lee was able to find an oral surgeon to do a root canal, and then a local dentist was more than willing to treat me after that. I also wondered if I should get my medical treatment out of town, to be sure my HIV status didn't reflect poorly on the kids. I didn't want them ostracized in any way because of what was happening to me.

Because I worried about transmitting the disease to the kids, Doug assured me—and everything I read confirmed it—that there had only been one confirmed case of casual transmission within a family. That case probably occurred because of the way a mother handled the diapers of her infected baby. If we would just observe common rules of cleanliness within the home, we should be fine, Doug said.

But how could I make five kids who loved to play Wrestlemania on Daddy understand that some of that was going to have to be toned down? Or how could I explain that they could only kiss me on the cheek now, and vice versa?

Not only that, how would I explain to them that I wouldn't be doing surgery anymore? Or, especially, how the same God we had so often credited with making them Rozars instead of orphans might one day allow them to become fatherless again? Who would take care of them? Would they have enough to live on? Would Donna have to sell the house? The list of unanswered questions seemed endless at first—mostly about the unknown and unknowable future.

When I took it one day at a time, I was better able to keep my life in perspective. Two days after starting AZT, for instance, we had a nice day in church, in spite of the malaise and nausea that was starting to develop from the medication. We took a pleasant family walk that evening, too. Later that night, as I put Jonathan Edward to bed, we recited the books of the Bible together and then I sang him the Lord's Prayer.

Jonathan Edward, who was then six, was really the only child old enough to begin to comprehend what was happening. One morning I took him out for breakfast, and we had a long, long talk. I tried to explain that I was sick and wouldn't be able to do heart surgery anymore because I wouldn't want to risk making my patients sick when I was trying to help them.

But the little guy knew how much I loved surgery. "Won't they let you do even one more, Dad? Just one?" he asked.

I fought back the tears and tried to get past the lump in my throat. "No, son. Not even one. This sickness I have is pretty serious. In fact, it may someday take my life." I watched his face to try to read his reaction and didn't have to wait long. "Well, then, Dad," he said, "you should be happy, not sad, because if you die you'll be with Jesus!"

Kids can be so matter-of-fact! His insight cut right through the mental and emotional fog I was struggling with. Of course, he was right, even if he didn't understand all the implications of what he had just said. I smiled and gave him a big bear hug, thankful that God had brought him into my life.

But there were other times when I fought the tears and lost, especially in those first few weeks while we waited for the disability question and other financial matters to be resolved. Although I kept going to work, making rounds on any of my patients still in the hospital after surgery, after a couple of weeks I really didn't have much meaningful work to do. That, on top of the problems I was having with AZT, was probably the main cause of my first real weeping in a long, long time.

I was sitting in the office in the dark, feeling sick and self-pitying as I thought about the kids, about leaving them in the world without a father. Who would mold them, tell them about all the hazards out there? *What are you going to do, God? I do believe you're sovereign, but I need to know how this is going to work out.*

There was some Christian music playing on my little radio, as tears ran down my face. *Oh, God, I can't leave these kids. I don't want to leave them. You brought these children into my life—and now you're going to take me out of theirs? Although our home's not perfect, and I'm not a perfect dad, I want to see them grow up and get excited about life. Am I going to miss all that?*

Almost as quickly, I added, *God, I'm probably being selfish. But is it really selfish to want to be with them and see them get through high school and graduate? That would be such a great thing!*

I went around and around with that. I knew I needed to put my whole trust in the Lord, but I wondered what he was going to do. *I had* put my whole trust in the Lord, and he let this happen. Even when he saved me, he knew it was going to happen. Even before I was born! *Lord, when I was born, you knew all this was going to happen, yet you guided my path through all that foolishness as a youth, and you brought me this far. So, Lord, I have to believe you know what you're doing.*

As a rule, surgeon types don't cry too often, either because of our training and everything we've experienced in terms of life and death and blood and gore, or maybe because that's just the way we are. This episode in the office was new to me, I assure you. Maybe it had something to do with the fact that without the clear-cut role I had had all these years, I didn't really know who I was anymore.

It's strange, but I wasn't worried that somebody would walk in on me. This was a private matter between God and me. Although I sometimes was tempted to think I had been abandoned, I always felt that he was there with me. Actually, I think—as a part of me—he was helping me release some of my emotions.

In that sense, my situation was a good thing. I was becoming acquainted with, and more honest about, other parts of myself, as if different layers of this former cardiac surgeon were being peeled away. I sometimes wondered whether there would still be anyone home when all the layers were peeled away.

One of the first layers to go was my personal privacy. Because I was a health-care worker, once my status became known, it was impossible to avoid public scrutiny, not only by my medical colleagues, but also by the Wisconsin Public Health Department, which by law had to investigate. The woman who interviewed me took what amounted to a "strip down" history. She wanted to probe into my life as far back as 1980. She was very persistent, grilling me for two hours about such matters as sexual promiscuity, homosexuality, and IV drugs.

When we started, I kept my guard up. But after she had asked all her questions without coming to any clear-cut conclusion—except that this case didn't fit the usual HIV profile—I had a chance to tell her how I was dealing with the illness. We even talked about the importance of faith in the face of this disease. When the interview was over, I think we had become pretty good friends.

Early on, I wasn't really talking to too many people about my diagnosis. But when the opportunity arose, I tried to express what I really believed. After my colleagues had been notified—without my knowledge and consent—one of them passed me in the hallway and kind of hung his head, without saying anything. I thought that was rather strange, since he had been so friendly up to that point. A half-hour later he returned, apologizing for not saying hello in the hall.

The issue of confidentiality is complex, especially in the health-care setting. My perspective, and that of my colleagues, may be different. However, the need for the clinic physicians and staff to know versus maintaining the privacy of our lives was an issue that never became that important. As we were always open about the situation, God's grace prevailed.

As we talked, I had an open door to tell this doctor how my faith was helping me through this crisis, that Jesus Christ had become my Sustainer. It was a really good conversation, the first specifically spiritual talk he and I had ever had. In the end, he said, "We're really going to miss you. I'm sorry this happened, and I certainly don't understand why. But let me know if I can do anything for you."

Moments like those pulled me up from the depths as I struggled to make sense of what was happening, and to discern what new directions God might have in mind for me. I was beginning to see how he could resurrect a significant ministry from the ashes of sorrow I was sitting in at that point in time. I began to hope that it wouldn't all be doom and gloom, and then the tomb. Could my God, who had overcome the tomb, help me overcome HIV, transforming my helplessness into helpfulness for someone else?

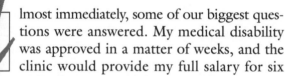

Dr. Rozar's Wild Ride

lmost immediately, some of our biggest questions were answered. My medical disability was approved in a matter of weeks, and the clinic would provide my full salary for six months. My medical care would be covered under the HMO, and if it ever was needed, the hospital's hospice would be available. The sizeable life insurance originally provided as part of my employee benefit package would be kept in effect.

Through it all, in spite of our fears, the Lord seemed to be saying, "How can you doubt my ability to take care of you in every detail?"

Although I didn't really have to work, I kept going to the office. It was partly through force of habit, but also my sense of obligation to do something doctor-like with my time as a way to repay the clinic's generosity. I had worked only about five months before I went on full disability on May 1, 1989.

Because I was used to working long hours, it seemed strange to be free—though I really was not. I couldn't put my career as a physician down. I had quit operating but everything in me resisted giving up being a doctor. For a while I still had some patients and patient families to care for, but I couldn't reveal anything about my own illness for fear of unnecessarily alarming them. Some of the cardiac-surgery patients would even stop by the office with a wound problem. I took care of them, though I didn't want to make that a habit.

Especially during May, I spent much of my "down time" in the office trying to sort things out, wrestling with occasional depression and sadness. Sometimes I would just sit at my desk, meditating, reading the Word, searching for some hope and help—and talking to the Lord, mostly about the kids. For a long time, I perceived this disease as more of a problem for them than it was for me.

Reading as many journal articles about HIV infection as I could put my hands on, it was easy enough to become resigned to an early, excruciating, slow death. On the other hand, I longed to stay around to help our children through adolescence, so much so that sometimes wishful thinking made me even question the diagnosis. Here I was, reading the awful facts about a disease I couldn't see, which had only become apparent through lab tests I never witnessed, done at a time when I had apparently been healthy. Once I even asked Doug, "Where is this thing?" When you're a surgeon, it's all the more difficult to become a prisoner of something you can neither see nor fix.

Why? HIV is a silent killer and you can get HIV without knowing it (as I did, or as Magic Johnson, Kimberly Bergalis, Arthur Ashe, or others have). Then, while you still feel healthy and appear healthy, you can transmit a disease worse than death to others—perhaps *many* others if you have sex with multiple partners or share contaminated needles while using IV drugs. There are other ways to get it, but these are the most common. "Innocent" victims (health-care workers, patients, and newborns) are also at risk from people with HIV, whether or not the diagnosis is known.

Yet, in spite of all the well-publicized warnings, some people are still risking acquiring HIV in exchange for a few minutes of pleasure. Are they betting that, as with so many other diseases, medicine will soon find a cure or even a vaccine for HIV? A vaccine may be developed someday, and I hope it is, so that those who are uninfected who insist on living an immoral lifestyle can be protected from their stupidity—at least from HIV infection. There is no vaccine, of course, to protect them from such other consequences as guilt, remorse, poor self-image, and the downward spiral where such activities inevitably lead.

A vaccine still won't help the millions of people already infected with HIV. And, from everything I've read and every informed person I've talked with, the possibility of a cure being found is still nearly zero. This is because of several things, including: (1) the way the virus attacks the immune system, incorporating itself into the DNA and then reproducing itself; and (2) the fact that it may mutate, once it has effectively taken over the immune system, making it harder to track down.

Nonetheless, the media seems ready to grasp any straw of hope the researchers toss out. I think this is mainly because if there is anything the children of the sex-and-pleasure revolution resist, it's returning to the only thing that could virtually eliminate AIDS within one generation—abstinence before marriage, and sexual faithfulness to one uninfected partner after marriage. Additionally, of course, IV drug abusers would have to either stop doing IV drugs or at least stop sharing needles.

For some time there was a lot of hype about the drug AZT being able to turn HIV disease into a manageable illness, like diabetes has become. I've taken AZT for a year, and it didn't have that effect for me.

These reports didn't mention that nothing available now (or even on the horizon) will tear down the wall of isolation that HIV infection builds, separating you sexually and in other ways from the people you love, and also from society, for the rest of your life. The fear of transmitting or acquiring HIV will exist until every HIV virus has been eradicated from an infected person's system. Even if that could be accomplished, could it be proven?

The material I studied graphically described how, generally speaking, AIDS patients die a horrible death, as infections and cancers that their body normally would fight off slowly sap their strength and vitality and finally take their lives. These diseases are called "opportunistic" because they take advantage of the opportunity provided by the person's compromised immunity to enter the body and make the person sick.

AIDS is called a "wasting" disease because it often kills people very slowly; in other words, they waste away. If you have observed this process in a person with AIDS, you know what I mean. Sometimes it has been made so public, nobody could miss it. This was true in the excruciating case of Kimberly Bergalis, who died in late 1991 after being infected through dental procedures. My own loss of twenty pounds in 1985 was another example. I've never been able to regain that weight, no matter how much food or how many calories I consume. I don't know why HIV disease has this effect, but perhaps it changes the body's metabolism in some fundamental way. There are whole villages of people in Africa—where AZT, acyclovir, and other high tech treatments may never be available—who are dying from "slim disease," as AIDS is known there.

Of all the horrifying possibilities I studied, the worst is called "dementia." Unlike many diseases, HIV can penetrate the central nervous system (CNS), so that a patient can slowly "lose his mind" while slowly losing his life. The idea of ending my life demented caused me the most concern. My own mother has been in a state of dementia for some time from Alzheimer's disease, and I have seen my kids' inability to relate to her in a meaningful way. They don't even want to touch her. I, like most HIV sufferers, would much prefer to die quickly, with my wits about me, than to have that one last impenetrable barrier erected between me and others, especially the little people I love so much.

As Donna and I both became AIDS-informed during those first few weeks after diagnosis—by reading and by watching videos—we discussed the question of "artificial" life-sustaining measures, should I become totally incapacitated. We agreed that despite how bad it might get, life would still be God's to give or take away, so I would always get food and water, even if it had to be administered artificially.

Believe me, although these are matters all spouses should discuss (and write out their wishes in that regard), just thinking about them in the context of my illness was subtly depressing. We did go so far as having a new will drawn up. We then decided that reading so much about AIDS and knowing so much medically about the "possibilities" wasn't really doing us that much good. It would be much better, emotionally, interpersonally, spiritually and even physically, to focus on more positive things.

Physically speaking, the treatment I received—AZT— proved far more troublesome than the disease itself. I kept trying to go to the office, but I was miserable; afflicted with dry skin and severe itching, anorexia, and general malaise. I was also constantly nauseated, with a terrible taste in my mouth. Maybe you've had that feeling: the combination of wanting to vomit but not being able to. I battled that constantly until I finally found an antidote: Coca Cola and lemon juice.

Those days were some of the hardest of my life. One evening, when I had stayed home all day because I was too weak and sick to do anything else, I was lying on the couch in our den, just off the kitchen, while everybody else was having supper. Suddenly, I was crying, feeling sorry for myself, and hoping that nobody would come in and see me like that. The radio was on, tuned to one of our local Christian stations. As I wept, the words of a song ministered to me: "He will not leave you this way." Embracing that thought, I gained new strength, dried my tears, went around the corner, and ate supper.

After I had been on AZT for about five weeks, we took a trip to Pennsylvania to visit relatives and do some sightseeing. It was during that trip that I hit the bottom. There I was, in somebody else's bed, sick, with no local physician to call on (maybe the local doctors would rather not get involved with HIV—you never know). The family was in and out every day, doing their own thing, having family reunions and a basic grand old time. But I couldn't join in because I had barely enough energy to get out of bed.

I had a fever, alternating between being hot and having chills with uncontrollable shaking—to the point where my teeth were chattering and I had cramps in my legs and soreness everywhere. I couldn't get out of bed and lie down on the sofa, just for a little change, because the house was full of people and I didn't want to bother them. I had stashed my private supply of liquids in the refrigerator, but I didn't want to take up too much room in there either. And if I had to use the bathroom, I didn't want to take too long because many other people needed access to it.

On top of all that malaise, I wondered what the relatives thought about my illness. Would they burn the mattress after we left? Were they afraid they might get HIV from the toilet seat, or from the dishes or utensils we shared—even though they had been washed? Were they mad I had dragged my family, and all of *them*, into what seemed like a stigmatized black hole?

It didn't help much, either, to read in the local papers while we were there about a fellow in his seventies who had just died of AIDS acquired through a blood transfusion during heart surgery. He had had a prolonged course of dying, and right after he died, his wife was diagnosed HIV-positive.

My personal agony (mostly physical, but emotional, too) got so bad that one day I said to the Lord, "If it's going to be like this, if I'm going to be this sick just from the medicine, not my primary illness, please either get it over with, or heal me. I don't think I can handle this anymore." I figured if I could get this sick just from the treatment, the disease itself was going to be far worse.

I would lie there thinking, *Things are backward here. This expensive medicine ($7,000.00 a year) is making me sicker.* Yet I was resigned to following my physician's advice. I had gone from being the doctor to being the patient, from being in control to being helpless, from being self-reliant to having to depend on somebody else's decisions and to follow his directions.

Maybe you're used to that, but I certainly was not, and I had no idea how dehumanizing being a patient can be. My role-reversal began the day I had to let somebody stick me for the test to confirm my HIV status. Since then, it's never changed, though my experience as a patient has had such ups and downs that if graphed, it would look like the stock-market curve. For a comparable experience, board the world's largest roller coaster or go to Disney World and take Mr. Toad's Wild Ride.

For about two months on AZT I really struggled, sliding lower all the time. Then all of a sudden in July, I woke up one morning and felt fine, super—no side effects, and lots of energy! I thought, *This is great! Now I can get on with my life.* I cut the grass, trimmed the trees, did all kinds of odd jobs that had gone undone for weeks.

Fairly soon, however, it became obvious that my bone marrow had stopped working. For about two weeks I had experienced a kind of "remission," but now if I was going to survive, I would have to have blood transfusions, regularly. It's one thing to have somebody stick you for a blood test, but entirely different to spend six to eight hours on your back while the IV drips somebody else's blood into your vein. Being a doctor made those days doubly difficult. The nurses, of course, knew me, and when they had to insert the IV, I think they were a little afraid of not getting it right in the first time. Maybe they were afraid of getting stuck themselves. I don't know. But even when what they were doing really hurt, I never let on.

On top of that, since it's a day-long procedure, I had to use the rest room from time to time. The image that really sticks in my mind to symbolize my role-reversal is Ed Rozar, M.D., pushing his IV pole into the bathroom, just like any other patient.

Once, when I was lying on the cot and getting a transfusion, one of the other doctors walked by the door. Although he glanced in, and I was sure he recognized me, he just kept right on going, without even stopping to say hello. Now that I was Patient Rozar, I guess he didn't know how to relate to me anymore. Because of HIV, there was now some invisible partition between us.

Donna happened to be with me that day, and it really teed her off, but I tried to help her understand that I wasn't offended, even if I was disappointed. Doctors are busy people, after all, and this man was one of the busiest. Later that day, while I was still being transfused (four units takes a long time) Donna met that fellow in the hallway. Since this time he couldn't escape, he mumbled something semi-apologetically about being awfully busy and hoping I would understand.

I don't think it was a lack of concern. And I couldn't really expect an outpouring of empathy, since I had been there only five months. Maybe my colleagues simply didn't know what to say. In fact, what can you say to a budding cardiac surgeon who all of a sudden can't operate anymore?

Besides Doug Lee, my physician, there was one other doctor who did reach out to me that summer—Scott Erickson, a six-foot-three internist who is at least as much at home in the boundary waters of Minnesota as he is in the Marshfield

Clinic. Scott knew just what this doctor-patient needed to get back on his feet—trout fishing!

When I say that, you probably envision an *Outdoor Life* calendar-type picture of a perfectly decked out angler, hip-deep in a crystal-clear mountain stream, calmly watching his perfectly placed dry fly settle over a waiting rainbow trout.

Unless, that is, you're familiar with Central Wisconsin fishing, where King Musky, Queen Walleye, and Prince Northern Pike rule over a piscatorial court comprised of panfish like the delicious crappie. Hardly anybody there takes brook-trouting seriously, for at least two reasons. First of all, the fish are generally fairly small—a twelve-inch native brookie is a monster! Besides, the beaver ponds and back-woods streams they inhabit are inaccessible to all but the most determined fishermen, who are undaunted by the swarms of hummingbird-sized mosquitoes that also inhabit the same locale.

Scott is that kind of fisherman, I discovered. The first time he led me through the cedar swamp to the Mecan River, I wondered what I had agreed to. We were at least a mile from nowhere, and I had spent a lot of money on waders. Believe it or not, the decision to spend that seventy-five dollars had been very hard to make, considering my prognosis. It better be worth it!

We weren't purists about it, either, choosing lightweight spinning gear and small spinners for bait. But even expert fisherman Lee Wulff couldn't have made a clean back cast with a fly rod in that swamp, where cedar, spruce, and poplar trees reached out from both sides of the ten-foot-wide creek to effectively canopy the creek throughout the year. Not infrequently, we would have to climb out and walk on the bank just to make progress upstream.

There was something about being out there, knee- to waist-deep in the gently flowing, slightly murky water, that was cleansing to the soul and the spirit. After a few minutes in that chilly stream, it was almost as if the cares of my world were swept away, erased by elements that had been flowing here since long before my troubles ever came to be. And they would still flow long after my troubles had been forgotten.

But there's a nibble! I sense it with my index finger, barely touching the four-pound-test monofilament line. *Let him take it. Don't set it yet!* My heart beats faster. *There!* I whip the rod tip upward with a wrist motion, and the five-foot light action rod bends as the trout rushes downstream, then upstream, then sideways, shaking its head to dislodge my hook until I gently slip my left hand under its belly.

I gaze at my prize for a moment, absorbed by the artistry of a ten-inch brook trout, its green and black mottled back just breaching the surface. Orange and yellow and purple dots decorate its heaving sides as I lift it higher, toward my creel. Now the bright orange belly comes in view. *This one is a native, no doubt,* I think, with a certain sense of accomplishment for having captured it. And then I see its delicate fins, nearly as colorful as a monarch butterfly—orange, with a black stripe in the middle and a white stripe along the leading edge.

Amazed at the unassuming yet intricate beauty of this creature, I reassure myself: *Another proof there is a God. How fortunate I am to know him, and even more to be known by him. Like this fish, my life is in his hand—or else this doctor is in deep, deep trouble.*

7

Life in Overdrive

truthfully now, what would you do if you thought you had only three years to live, maybe only one of them in reasonable health? That's not a bad question to ask yourself, even if you don't have a terminal illness. But it's totally different when you see it in black and white on a legal document. When you think you're dying, every day—maybe every issue—takes on a different sense of urgency.

When I started feeling well enough, we put our life into overdrive. I had agreed to retrain in a similar but noninvasive field of medicine, peripheral vascular studies. Compared to cardiac surgery, it wasn't much of a challenge, but it would give me some use for my M.D. degree, and I could continue serving the clinic in some way, at least for a while.

One of the secondary benefits of this decision was that in the fall of 1989 I was able to take the whole family with me to retrain. We drove first to Detroit in September, for a one-week course in vascular technology. A month later we drove to Seattle for more retraining, a three-week trip during which we visited some national parks, including Mount Rushmore, putting more than four thousand miles on the van. All this was on the heels of June's three thousand miles of traveling to Pennsylvania to visit family and a trip to northern Minnesota for a church family camp over Labor Day weekend.

Throughout this period, I was getting transfusions every three or four weeks. In all, I've received more than thirty units of blood—like some kind of medical vampire! In fact, we had to stagger the trips to allow for the transfusions.

We were driven people, trying to beat my doctor's estimate that I might only live until 1992. So we squeezed three or four years of family activities into one—just in case. Not that we sat around the table saying, "Wouldn't it be wise to run ourselves ragged this year because Dad might not be able to travel next year?" But, interestingly enough, when we stopped to take photos, Donna often volunteered to work the camera so I could be in the picture.

One other factor in all these travels was that they took me away from Marshfield to places where people didn't know me and where I wasn't reminded daily of what I was missing. This tension was mainly internal, since nobody in Marshfield pressured me about the illness. But had I been at home, I would have felt obligated to go to work, where I would have seen all the heart and thoracic surgeons coming and going, busier than ever—without me.

If you want to identify with me, just think of something you really love to do—jog, cycle, play tennis, bingo or shuffleboard, fish or hunt with your buddies, or participate in a quilting bee—whatever. Now imagine you've had a stroke. How would you feel, sitting there in a wheelchair, watching, listening to all the friendly chatter and banter you used to relish so much. Give that feeling a name, and you're getting close to where I was, because operating was my life.

"Disappointment" is close, but mix in some "emptiness" and "frustration," too. It felt like part of my life was gone, as if somebody sneaked into the kitchen overnight and cut out a piece of the pie. Only now that I couldn't bake another pie, the missing part was irreplaceable.

Looking back on those rather frenetic few months, maybe the process of having my layers peeled away had reached the father/husband level. I wanted so much to give the kids as many happy memories as we could fit into whatever time we had left together, even if they were a little young to really appreciate some of the things we did.

One thing's for sure, though: Thinking I was dying helped me appreciate my family more than ever before. Now, almost more than anything else, I wanted to see us become a close-knit, loving, caring unit, committed to common principles and goals.

Being a surgeon is like being in many other professions or jobs—in the sense that you go in early, work hard all day, and get home twelve to fourteen hours later, exhausted. When you're in that mode, the family just sort of goes along on its own track while you concentrate on being their provider. Before my illness, I hadn't been an integral part of the family during the week. I simply wasn't home most of the time! And even when I *was* there, I had a beeper on, and the telephone could ring at any moment, so it was nearly impossible to be totally at home and not partly somewhere else.

Once I began to stay home more, I began to see more clearly what family life was supposed to be like—a 24-hour-a-day involvement, not just from 6:00 P.M. to 10:00 P.M. I developed a new perspective on the children, especially how they could minister to me, and me to them. Our relationships became more important, and my role as a father, rather than primarily as a breadwinner, became more pressing. I began to fully appreciate Donna's role as a mother and "nurturer" of the family. I became far more focused on building into our kids the kind of character and discipline they would need to carry on without me. That was one of the biggest pressures I felt, as if I could somehow condense parenthood, protecting them from temptations that they wouldn't really face for years.

I probably I was too hard on them, too intense, an over-reaction complicated by the fact that I was around them more, so I knew what was going on. On top of that, especially when I was taking AZT, I wasn't feeling good. I might be nauseated, for instance, just when they wanted to turn my bed into a trampoline—with me on it! They didn't understand the situation, and I was sometimes too demanding and impatient.

But that was more than irritability from being sick. I felt that if I didn't control them now, how would they learn? If they didn't learn discipline and respect from their father now, it might never happen. So, if they were being disrespectful, acting up, or not eating well at the table, I not only focused on their present actions, but also on what they might become if they didn't shape up. I tried to explain, "I want you to grow up to be godly boys and girls, to respect your elders, to obey and control yourselves. I may not be here later to teach you, so I want you to learn now."

In reality, my approach was unfair to them. I pushed too hard. I tried to make them grow up too fast. Before I became sick, I figured—like most parents—that I would have time later to help them develop and mature.

Donna and I had our share of conflict about this. Having me around the house all day long made her life much more difficult in many ways. Now there was one more person to think about, especially when I was sick. It was more an expression of her love than I realized at the time that she generally put up with my expectations and demands. But once in a while, when I was being unreasonable or at least unrealistic in terms of the kids, she would remind me, "Just let them be children, Ed. They can't be adults yet. If we push too hard, we might win the battle but lose the war later."

My dilemma was that I had to relinquish what I as a doctor prized most—control. In terms of my family's future, and even my own, the outcome was in the hands of God, not mine. I had become God's patient, and he my heart surgeon, sitting on my hospital bed, drawing on the sheets, trying to help me understand what he was going to do. More importantly, he wanted me to trust him.

I don't know if I was a good patient or a difficult one. But I do know that, once we got past the initial large hurdles about finances, I spent a lot of energy trying to understand what this illness meant. What could be done about it? What had God said about it in his Word? Where was I, from his point of view? What was his perspective?

I began to seriously search the Scriptures, looking for every possible promise to claim, every case similar to mine, every message my Divine Healer might be trying to communicate to his twentieth-century patient. I read voraciously because I was hungry to learn not only what he said in his Word, but more importantly, how to know him better, to get as close to God as one human being could possibly get.

I had read the Bible through at least three times before, but this time through it seemed to come alive. It was more real, more relevant, more practical. I was learning that the Word of God really is "living and active and sharper than any two-edged sword, and piercing as far as the division of soul and spirit . . . able to judge the thoughts and intentions of the heart" (Heb. 4:12).

In the Book of Job, I found a kindred spirit, adopting his policy of not charging God with wrongdoing, although, like Job, I had many questions and only a few answers. I concurred with him, a man perhaps even more afflicted than I, that, "He knows the way I take; When He has tried me, I shall come forth as gold" (Job 23:10). And I affirmed his trust: "Though He slay me, I will hope in Him . . ." (Job 13:15).

Hundreds of other passages nurtured my soul during those days, slowly pumping strength into my weakness, as if I were receiving a spiritual transfusion. I could almost hear God whispering, as he did to the apostle Paul, "My grace is sufficient for you, for power is perfected in weakness" (2 Cor. 12:9). And I echoed Paul's declaration: "Therefore I am well content with weaknesses, with insults, with distresses . . . with difficulties, for Christ's sake; for when I am weak, then I am strong" (v. 10).

The prophet Isaiah spoke directly to my situation, "Behold, God is my salvation, I will trust and not be afraid. For the LORD GOD is my strength and song" (Isa. 12:2). Also in the Book of Isaiah was a story so like my own that it seemed to be a message straight from God. "In those days Hezekiah became mortally ill. And Isaiah . . . came to him and said to him, Thus says the LORD, 'Set your house in order, for you shall die and not live'" (Isa. 38:1).

But when Hezekiah cried out to God for mercy, he received an additional fifteen years of life. Would he do the same for me? Did I dare to ask? Why not? Our God is the same yesterday, today, and forever. So I prayed, very specifically, for twelve more years, long enough to see my oldest son through high school. I thought, *If I can just stay around and help him mature until he gets through high school, then he can become the leader in the family and help take care of things.* Of course, I wanted to see all my children grow up. I suppose, by my human nature I would have asked for more after the twelve years were over.

The more I immersed myself in the Word, the more I discovered that the coin of affliction has two sides. Every testing is also a hidden opportunity to show that our faith is real; more than that, to prove—to others as well as ourselves—that *God* is real.

My first major presentation on the topic of AIDS was at a special conference in June 1990 in Wheaton, Illinois, sponsored by the Christian Medical and Dental Society. But before I tell you what I said, I need you to understand that getting up in front of any crowd, much less an assembly of my peers, to discuss something as intensely personal as my HIV status and all its implications is not something that the old Ed Rozar would have wanted to do. But once I started working on my presentation, I had more trouble figuring out what to leave out than what to say. I had so much I wanted to discuss, not so much about AIDS as a disease, but about how God could turn such an apparent tragedy into an opportunity for ministry.

I wanted to exhort my colleagues to stop and take stock of their lives *before they were forced to do so.* If they were at all like me before diagnosis, their whole lives were planned all the way through retirement. Had they considered that God might have something totally different in store? It's so easy for physicians to think we are the masters of our own destinies—potters instead of clay—and this may be even more common among surgeons, who so often function like mini-potters: rebuilding, reworking, rearranging. Surgery is an awesome vocation, but it's just too easy to let success ruin your sense of humility.

Putting that talk together was a real turning point for me. I had to solidify my thinking about such basic things as: Who is God, really? What is he like? What are his promises? I spent days on that program, wrestling, redoing, adding new stuff almost right up to the time I spoke. But, during that sorting process, my hunger for truth—and for God, who *is* that truth—intensified. When I finally got it organized to my satisfaction, the talk, which included slides, was infused with Scripture, almost forty references in just a few pages.

I wanted to be crystal-clear that my hope and courage did not come from myself, but from God and his Word. Left to myself, I could never have found the right perspective. But I did find it in Psalm 39:

LORD, make me to know my end,
  And what is the extent of my days,
  Let me know how transient I am.
Behold, Thou hast made my days *as* handbreadths,
  And my lifetime as nothing in Thy sight,
  Surely every man at his best is a mere breath.
  (vv. 4–5)

I wanted to open some eyes and hearts to the implications of this plague and to call for compassion from my colleagues. I hoped the message would hit home: that my disease is real, and what happened to me could happen to anyone. I wanted them to realize it was time to get involved, to reach out and touch people with AIDS the way Jesus touched the lepers of his day. I had needed my illness to change my attitude toward HIV-positive folks, to see them as creations of God. Maybe I could save someone else the agony of learning the same lesson the same way.

AIDS patients are on the threshold of eternity. They are lonely people who often don't have the support of family or friends. It's a tremendous opportunity to minister, but one has to stop and take the time. I told my audience they had to be there and listen, though it's difficult to reach out when there's nothing more to be done medically and there are so many other patients to care for.

Since they were physicians, I told them about my symptoms and treatments and the challenge of becoming a patient. During my first year after diagnosis, my T4-cell count had fallen from 230 (normal is 1,000) to 30. I described the effects of AZT, and the failure of erythropoietin injections to stimulate my bone marrow. After three weeks of extremely painful injections, I was glad it had failed. With the dropping T4-cell count, we started a monthly treatment of pentamadine. "I don't know if you've ever taken inhalation therapy," I said, "but the plastic by itself tastes awful, and pentamadine is extremely bitter." I reminded them that many doctors aren't really aware of the side effects, dehumanization, and outright discomfort their patients experience when they follow their physician's orders.

I described other medical details, too. In April of that year, yeast began growing in my mouth—a very frightening experience! I ignored it the first time, but then it came back. A week later I had developed such a severe cough that it would wake me up at night, and I wondered if I was going to end up with a hernia. I dragged my feet about getting an X-ray, until Donna called Doug and I had to admit what was going on. We looked at the films together, and there was pneumonia all right, but probably not pneumocystis.

Because I was on AZT for HIV, Nizoral for the yeast, and Doxycycline for the pneumonia, sometimes I felt like a walking pharmacy! Donna seemed more concerned about my pneumonia than I was. She even asked me if I was disappointed. "About what?" I replied.

"It looks like it's started," she said. "When's your first bronchoscopy?" Both of us, at that point, were prepared for the worst, a gradual decline, probably marked by numerous pulmonary problems. I told the audience I had thought about what was coming, too. I was going to get the oldest pulmonary specialist in the clinic to do the procedures, rather than a young guy. That way, if he got infected, it wouldn't seem quite so bad. That may have been a crazy way of thinking, but I was really concerned about spreading this disease.

My first presentation was well received, but if I gave it today, I would try to communicate a simple but profound lesson I'm still learning. It goes something like this:

> Friends, there is more. There is more to life than being a physician who happens to be a believer. Sometimes we modify the word *Christian* with adjectives like "sincere," "born-again," "devout," or even "Spirit-filled." But that's just window dressing. A Christian is a Christian. A Christian physician is a Christian who happens to be a physician.

There is more to faith than Sunday school and church and rushing home to see the ball game on TV. We need to get serious about who God is, and what he desires for us and requires of us. He's not the "man upstairs," or the "big guy." He is the Creator—*our* Creator. He is our Father—Abba, Father—in reality, he's our loving Daddy. He wants us to be whole in him, no matter what the circumstances. He requires our faithful obedience even when the actions involved might seem illogical, impractical, or worse.

In the same way, there is more to marriage and family life than being a good provider and taking everybody on nice vacations while accepting relational mediocrity as "good enough." A Christian has the opportunity and responsibility to "press on" for everything God desires for him or her.

My priorities were rearranged for me through this crisis. Will it take that to rearrange your own to the point where you earnestly seek his will *before* going ahead, instead of asking him to bless your decisions *after* they're made?

I would conclude a talk with this challenge: "Examine your foundations, now! Once the storm begins, you'll be so occupied with it that you won't be able to get underneath and shore up the weak spots." (This revelation truth came from one of Pastor Glenn Smith's messages as associate pastor of Believers' Church. I have used this example many times in impressing on people that only with the Lord is one's future secure. And I would echo an unknown author's words, printed in *Our Daily Bread:* "I thank you Lord for bitter things; they've been a friend of grace; they've driven me from paths of ease, to seek the Father's face."

When I finished that June 1990 conference, I was exhausted and exhilarated at the same time. At the close of my talk, perhaps a hundred of my colleagues gathered at the front of the auditorium to pray for me. It was the first time I felt so affirmed, accepted, and supported. More significantly, though, an important change was taking place within me.

Until my diagnosis, I had thought my mission was to be a cardiac surgeon. Then, from the day I put down the instruments until that conference, I had lacked a real sense of direction. But being there was like turning the page to the beginning of a new chapter. Or, to use another analogy, it felt as if the dark clouds were being blown away and the sunshine was coming through. All of a sudden I saw a new horizon I hadn't imagined—a vista dotted with people needing to hear a voice of faith and hope in the midst of this epidemic, whether they were patients, their families, or health-care workers.

When I thought about it, I realized that instead of being near the end of something, I was at the beginning of a new adventure. Who better to carry this message to physicians, legislators, and lay people—and all Christians? I could look at AIDS from both sides, patient and health-care worker, without a hidden agenda or a self-serving motivation.

I wanted to tell the whole truth about AIDS because I knew that facts would ultimately overrule both hysteria and self-interest. It was obvious to me that good science, good medicine, good public policy and good AIDS education must either be built on truth or be bankrupt (and in this case, lethal).

Yet, as my willingness to speak out became more broadly known, I discovered that not everyone was happy to hear me say that with this disease, as with any disease, it is always better to know where we stand than to be uninformed and risk the consequences. Knowledge, not ignorance, had become a focal point in my way of looking at HIV—and I hoped it would be that way for others.

God was showing me that the last and greatest adventure in life was not dying, but living. The fire within me was started by a tiny spark. Over the next year and a half, it would become a roaring blaze, fed by the Word of God and the prayers of his people.

8

Hype, Hysteria, and Hope

*i*n terms of my illness, the rest of 1990 was pretty quiet, but I kept giving my presentation in both medical and lay settings as the opportunities came along. In July 1991, however, the whole thing exploded. Several articles appeared in major medical publications, and we received local and national newspaper coverage. After that, it wasn't long before Donna and I were sitting in the "green room" of NBC's "Today" show.

Here's how it happened. I had participated in an AIDS panel in May at the Marshfield Clinic, where I simply stated the facts as well as my beliefs. In the midst of the discussion, I said, "We've been talking a lot about the disease, but not one thing has been said yet about sex. Let's clear the air. When AIDS began, 80 to 90 percent of the people involved were homosexuals. Most of the rest were IV drug abusers and bisexual men."

Now, if you want to get some mail or phone calls, that's all you have to say. I was accused of gay-bashing, being homophobic (whatever that is) and proselytizing—because I had also shared how my faith was sustaining me.

However, there was such good response to the honest and open discussion that the clinic offered the panel again, and this time the media came. Not much new was said but we did touch on some pressing problems. Interestingly enough, all the media interviews that day focused on a homosexual on the panel who had lost his job and whose lover had already died of AIDS. It irked me a bit, but I recall praying, "Lord, that's fine. If they don't want to interview me, so be it."

But the next thing I knew, TV Channels 7 and 9 from Wausau came down on separate days to interview and tape me for their news programs. That same week a crew from Channel 11 in Minneapolis traveled here to do a segment on my situation. These were pleasant experiences, and I was more than glad to be involved. At that same time, there was a big flap in Minneapolis about two local HIV-positive physicians.

A week later, when I was at a summer fishing camp with Jonathan Edward, NBC-TV was calling, as well as CBS. Channel 11 (an NBC affiliate) had sent a clip of my interview to New York, and the network had aired it Friday morning, July 12. The initial Centers for Disease Control (CDC) proposal on HIV testing for health-care workers was due to be released, and they wanted both Donna and me to appear in person and as soon as possible. CBS would interview me the same day and show it as a live interview the next morning.

I have to be candid with you: Flying into New York and being treated like celebrities was like a fairy tale. We were met at the airport by a big, black limo that took us to a very nice hotel. A team from a Pittsburgh TV station was waiting for us—trying to scoop the others, I suppose—but we didn't give them an interview because we wanted to honor our first commitment to NBC. The next morning, when we headed for the studio at 6:15, the Pittsburgh cameraman was waiting in the lobby. So we got filmed going to another limo. *Big deal*, I would have thought, had I seen that on the nightly news. But being there was a totally different matter.

Now I'm going to tell you a trade secret—at NBC the "green room" (where you wait to be next on camera) is actually green! At CBS, it's a different color even though they still call it the "green room." I have been told that this phrase comes from Shakespearean times when the actors would wait in the green shrubbery before going on stage.

Faith Daniels did the interview for the "Today" show, and she was super. Nobody mentioned that the CDC director, Dr. William Roper, would appear just before us from the Washington, D.C., studio. That was a little ironic, since if the CDC and others charged with disease control had taken HIV seriously enough at first, I might never have been infected.

NBC's studio is beautiful, with wood paneling and inlaid marble and lights and cameras everywhere. There are actually three sets side by side: one for the opening, one for news, and the third, where we waited on the sofa, more informally decorated, like a living room.

After a short introduction of my HIV history, Faith began the interview by asking, "Was there ever any question in your mind what you would choose to do [after diagnosis]?" I responded with the fact that I stopped operating as a cardiac surgeon because I felt it was the moral and ethical thing to do. She went on to ask what I thought about the new CDC guidelines requiring more patient and health-care worker testing, and what I thought the answer to the HIV problem was as far as physicians go. I said I felt that the guidelines did not go far enough, but that I was encouraged by their appearance, and as far as our profession was concerned, I was hopeful that we would be able to police ourselves.

For some reason, I wasn't nervous, maybe because I had been doing similar interviews for a few months. Donna seemed a little more tense with it all, but she did very well, nonetheless. Ms. Daniels spoke directly to Donna's heart: "Donna, it must have had a tremendous effect on you and the children." Donna responded that many positive things had happened and that there had been abundant opportunities to share where our hope comes from.

In fact, our interview was going so well, it was continued after the break. Faith made a very profound statement how ironic it was that physicians, whose mission was to save lives, could put their patients at risk. At the end, Faith said, "Your courage is inspiring," but I don't know exactly what she meant. Maybe she was thinking of my positive attitude toward my illness, or about wanting to express my views instead of hiding in a closet and waiting to die. However, if she was thinking about my point that health-care workers doing invasive procedures owe it to themselves and their patients to know their HIV status, and to retrain if it is positive, I don't see that as courageous. I was just stating what is obviously the right thing to do.

Before we knew it, the interview was over, and we were off in the limo to CBS, where Paula Zahn taped an interview of us for a program to air the next day. The studios there are comparable to NBC's, with the exception that in the "holding room," people can watch monitors that are tuned to their competitors.

Although the basic stuff Paula wanted to cover was similar to what we had talked about at NBC, she built on it a little. After our introduction and a brief summary of our situation, she wanted to go deeper. "We've got two stories here," she said, but there wouldn't be enough time to fully discuss our personal story as well as the ramifications for my profession.

We covered questions ranging from patients' rights and my opinion of the CDC guidelines, to whom Donna "blamed" for my infection. Paula did make a very interesting comment early in the interview following my comment that the CDC guidelines were overdue: "If doctors had any inkling at all that they carried the virus, they should quit doing surgery."

The fast-paced world of sound-bites and quick-fixes can't adequately explore the multifaceted plight of an HIV-positive, born-again former cardiac surgeon, his wife, and their family. I don't want to seem ungrateful; it's just the reality of TV news coverage. Everybody, from the limo drivers to the makeup people to the interviewers, treated us like royalty. One of the funny things was that the CBS segment of Health Watch was sponsored by a denture adhesive: "Orafix really sticks." I hope that our message "stuck" as firmly with the TV viewers.

By evening, we were home in Wisconsin again, and the interviews almost seemed like a dream, except for the message on my answering machine to call Dr. Bill Roper. And the next day, there we were on the tube on the CBS "This Morning" program. For average Americans, this was heavy stuff.

After that, the dike broke, and we were overwhelmed with so many requests for interviews, panel appearances, and the like, that the whole summer of 1991 was a blur.

We flew to Pittsburgh, where my story was front-page news for some time. Here we were, chauffeured around again, this time in a white stretch limo. I'll never forget Donna saying, "I could get used to this!" I just smiled back and said, "Don't." But I was glad she was enjoying herself.

In Pittsburgh we did an hour-long, live TV talk show, "Pittsburgh Talking," on WTAE, during which I had total freedom to talk about anything. Adam Lynch did the show, and it was a rewarding experience. I knew there were people there from the Pittsburgh Academy of Medicine, and the director of surgery at one of the hospitals was appearing with us.

But I was more nervous about a particular guy in the audience. He wasn't dressed very well, and he had a long earring hanging off one ear. *He's a plant,* I figured. *He'll try to drag us off into the homosexuality smokescreen, for sure.* When the time came for questions from the audience, however, I learned a big lesson about prejudging people when he asked, "Dr. Rozar, can you tell me how your faith has sustained you through all this?"

Adam Lynch started the show with the statement that "for the last several weeks, only Barry Bonds and President Bush have had more publicity on Pittsburgh television." The reason was that Pittsburgh is most likely where I got infected, and the hospital where it happened was very unhappy with all the notoriety and interest in the situation.

More public appearances followed, and in August we appeared on "The 700 Club." Both Donna and I came away with the impression it hadn't gone nearly as well as in the secular setting. Maybe it was because Pat Robertson's first comment was, "You don't look so bad!" Normally, I would take that as a compliment, but it goes right to the heart of the whole problem with HIV transmission. Often, people who are infected *don't look so bad*. In fact, they can look pretty good. Too good. Ask Magic Johnson and Arthur Ashe.

Overall, it just seemed like Pat and I were not on the same wavelength. He wanted to talk about testing, the public-health officials "deceiving" us, and "this homosexual lobby," who were to blame for bringing this plague on themselves and us. I tried to buffer that, to show him it wasn't just a homosexual disease. But isn't it ironic that on a major Christian TV program I felt obliged to say this? Why? Because anti-homosexuality convictions (which is consistent with Scripture) have kept many conservative Christians from thinking clearly about HIV.

I did have to do some educating during the segment with Pat Robertson, but the Lord blessed the time, and the Holy Spirit gave me wisdom. Looking at the tape later, it seemed to have come off very well.

I used to be confused about the homosexuality issue myself, until I realized that the list of "bad people" in the world begins with me. It is just as unrighteous (or self-righteous) for the uninfected to make light of this disease (and people who have it) as it is for those who acquire AIDS by violating God's moral laws! To me, the logic is clear enough, even without bringing in the drug abusers, hemophiliacs, children, and others, including health-care workers like me, who have acquired AIDS in some other way. That is not to say that we shouldn't do all we can to protect others. For instance, on August 23, I had a chance to address the CDC in Atlanta, the primary agency responsible for developing guidelines to contain HIV within the health-care community. Although the CDC has no regulatory power, its guidelines are usually enacted into law by the various states and federal statutes. Their proposals had just come out, so it was an ideal time to say I thought the statement was too weak, and why. There were maybe twenty to twenty-five people present, and they were cordial enough, even if I was disputing their guidelines. Maybe they let me say my piece because for once they were not being blasted by an activist. Here was a "real person" who happened to get pulled into the AIDS debate through no choice of his own, except to retrain in surgery at precisely the wrong time.

It was exciting to meet some key players in our national strategy to combat this plague—people I had been reading about for years. They wanted to know how I was dealing with the illness, how I got it, what I thought about health-care workers with this disease, mandatory testing, and the new CDC guidelines. These guidelines suggested that health-care workers involved with invasive procedures should know their HIV status. If positive, they should withdraw from doing invasive procedures, unless a peer-group panel decided they could continue. Continuing, however, would require the informed consent of their patients.

I said they should be more stringent, more clear-cut regarding do's and don'ts, instead of "what if's." I didn't think the panel idea was enough. In my opinion, an HIV-positive surgeon should do something else, period. There is no good reason to compromise on that. It's the right thing to do.

"The American public doesn't trust you," I said. "They perceive the CDC as not taking the ball with this thing in the 1980s, and this is the time, with these guidelines, to reinstill public trust [and physician trust] in the CDC. The problem is, right now, everybody who's HIV-positive is hiding, fearful they might lose their jobs once their HIV status becomes known. So there has to be a safety net to catch these folks. Otherwise we're going to drive them further underground."

HIV infection is an extremely complex health issue, probably like no other in history, yet the variety of groups interested in this disease is truly amazing. I finally realized that many of the agendas and so-called solutions are based on wrong motivation and/or misinformation. When I became acquainted with Americans For A Sound AIDS/HIV Policy (A.S.A.P.), I began to see what role I could play in helping inform the public. Later, I accepted an invitation to be on their advisory board. Shepherd Smith, the president of A.S.A.P., had asked me if I would testify before a congressional committee on a bill regarding more diagnosis of HIV. The initial date was cancelled for political reasons. We were told that a room was not available for the hearing. Were those politicians who were against HIV testing hoping that Kimberly Bergalis would die before the hearing?

However, on September 26, 1991, I addressed the congressional hearing on what has been referred to as the Kimberly Bergalis bill. Kimberly Bergalis was one of the patients infected by her dentist in Florida. The bill would require testing of health-care workers and patients. I'll never forget walking into that austere hearing room, with the congressmen on the committee sitting up there above us, and all the media people filling the room behind us. The main thing that struck me was the sense of an evil presence there. There was something not quite right about the whole atmosphere.

When Kimberly Bergalis was wheeled into the room, there was an explosion of flashbulbs, and a near-hysterical frenzy among the press. Kimberly looked somewhat refreshed, but was obviously very compromised physically. She made her statement, which lasted only about twenty seconds, but will probably stick in the mind of anyone who saw her. Then her father, George Bergalis, spoke. This confrontation had the appearance of Custer's Last Stand.

Originally, this hearing was supposed to be just for people who favored the bill, but its opponents (mainly Democrats) had managed to postpone the proceedings. After the Bergalis's testimony about six people gave the opposing side. It was the same old nonsense: "We can't afford testing." "It won't make any difference." "What do we need to test for?" "What are we going to do with HIV-positive health-care workers?" "Aren't alcoholic and drug-abusing doctors more dangerous?"

One thing that seemed significant to me was that after George and Kimberly Bergalis left, all the Republican committee members left, too, except for California Republican William Dannemeyer, sponsor of the bill. He stayed the whole time. Many of the Democratic committee members stayed and gave unsupported, negative comments about the bill. Evidently many congressmen had already made up their minds before the hearing even began, but they needed the kind of media exposure that would portray them as concerned about the rights of the uninfected. It burned me up to see those guys leave. Not only did I believe what I had to say was important, but I had traveled at my own expense, interrupting a family vacation to be there.

But I gave about a five-minute statement anyway, which went something like this:

> This is a medical disease that I know a lot about personally, since I'm HIV-positive from doing surgery. This is not primarily a question of civil rights, as if AIDS deserves such status.
>
> In medical school, the very first principle we're taught is *primum non nocere*, Latin for "first of all do no harm." That's why I quit doing invasive procedures and got retrained in

another medical field. Once I knew my own HIV status, the only right thing to do was to avoid putting any patients at risk; even one is too many. We hear all kinds of statistics about what chance there is of reverse transmission. But even one in a million is too high, especially when that one person is you.

We are wallowing in a sea of ignorance, by our own choice. It's almost as if we don't want to know. That's dumb, but it's been a consistent perspective from the beginning. When you link that with selfish motives among both high-risk groups and physicians, you have a full-blown disaster. That's how we got where we are. When are we going to do something about it?

Putting blinders on—or keeping them on—won't solve anything, for the doctor or the patient or the general public. There is no other disease where we act as though we prefer that patients not know their status. In the history of plagues, there has never been, until now, a communicable disease the carriers of which were protected by the law. It would have been irrational then, and is irrational now. To spend billions of money on AIDS research without including the starting point of diagnosis through testing is absurd.

My testimony was over before I knew it. The opposing view was stated by Dr. Hacib Aoun, who had been infected from a broken lab vial and then kicked out of his training program. In spite of his own history, he said, "We don't need testing. HIV-infected workers can continue working as usual."

Although I didn't want to destroy Dr. Aoun, I made the point that he was not a surgeon, nor had he ever practiced surgery, so he had no idea of the degree of risk for either a health-care worker or a patient. His theory might sound nice but it is unrealistic. Surely he and others must know that "universal precautions" cannot be followed 100 percent of the time.

I felt the trip was worth taking, even though the bill failed, mainly because it was opposed by certain special-interest groups, including the American College of Surgeons and other groups of people who don't like anybody telling them what to do. For one thing, I wanted to support the Bergalis family. Together we visited the White House, where the Bush administration chose to totally ignore us. The reason for that is unclear, but I suspect it was politically motivated. While I was in Washington I also visited the Family Research Council and spoke at the Concerned Women of America national meeting.

The Bush administration was not the only group to distance itself from those who support HIV testing. CNN's "Crossfire" program cancelled an interview they had tentatively scheduled. That was okay with me, but George Bergalis, who was to appear with me, refused to be a guest when he learned I had been unfairly excluded. Maybe the whole thing was an answer to prayer, because by that time I was pretty beat and just needing to get back to my family.

Although other opportunities to present my views became available, they were generally oriented toward conflict and confrontation. The Oprah Winfrey show, for instance, wanted me to appear, but I knew that if certain activists were on stage or in the crowd, they might transform discussion of a serious public health issue into a civil rights circus. The issues involved are far too important to let them get obscured by media hype or special-interest group chicanery.

One invitation we did accept, however, was from ABC's "20/20," because the format of the show would be less combative and on our own turf. In November they sent a crew of five production people, the producer, Diane Forbes, and Lynn Sherr to Marshfield. Filming was done first at the clinic and then at our home, where the actual interview was held. It was easier to express ourselves, even to *be* ourselves, in this kind of format.

I will never forget Lynn's reaction when we got to the house, which they had totally rearranged to shoot those forty-five seconds that you may have seen on January 31, 1992. Here was this beautiful but somewhat stern woman who had interviewed many people, saying, "Where are the kids? I hope they'll be around." In fact, when the kids showed up, the whole thing lightened up. At the end they had our whole family walk down the street holding hands. We haven't done that in a million years! We usually look like a herd of cows when we go for a walk—three or four out front and a couple more bringing up the rear, with the dog in between.

I think what impressed Lynn most was hearing me say: "You know, life is so great! We don't have to crawl in a hole and give in to this disease. We can still choose to live every day, one at a time, as fully as possible, with God's help."

She asked me many questions and the answers came easily. In fact, she said, "This was great! Just great!" Yet—because the team spent several hours at the clinic and three to four at the house—we were surprised to see how little they used. The issue of HIV infection in health-care workers was never really addressed. I would not have taken the time or energy had I known that it would be such a one-sided presentation. Although I disagree with the viewpoint that opposes testing and retiring HIV-infected health-care workers, I am willing to hear them out. The public needs more open discussion and arbitration, not reporting that reflects bias and limited information.

One of our favorite programs was done for "Physicians Journal Update," which airs on the Lifetime cable network. Filming was done at the clinic and at our home. The real issues were addressed, and they also included our personal side. I suspect the audience that viewed it was already convinced of the need for more "routine" testing and practice modification for HIV-infected health-care personnel.

David Biebel

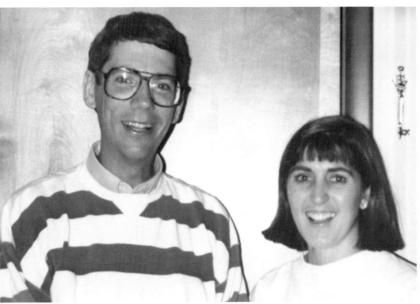

Ed and Donna, 1991

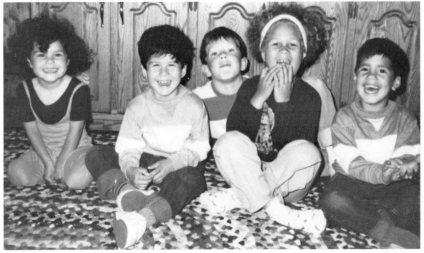

Christina, Jonathan Wayne, Jonathan Edward, Victoria, David, 1989

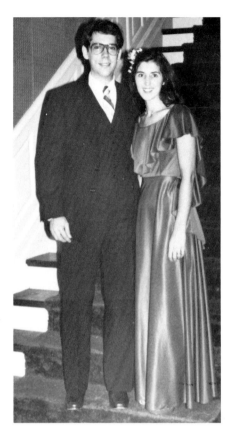

1980

Surgery in Ghana,
West Africa

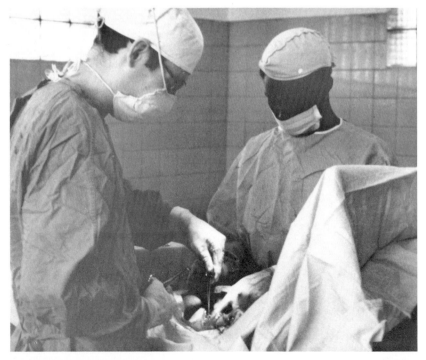

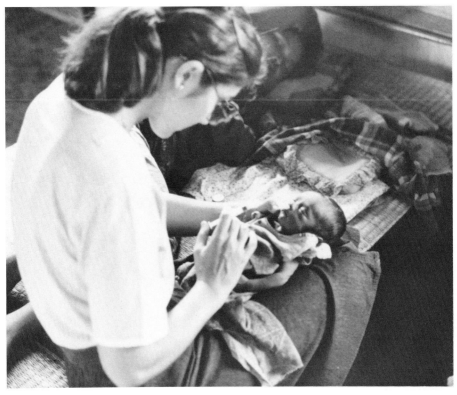

Serving in Thailand refugee camp 1982

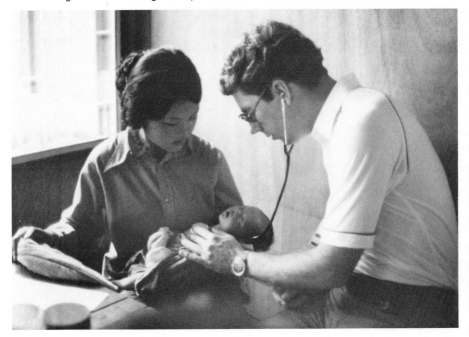

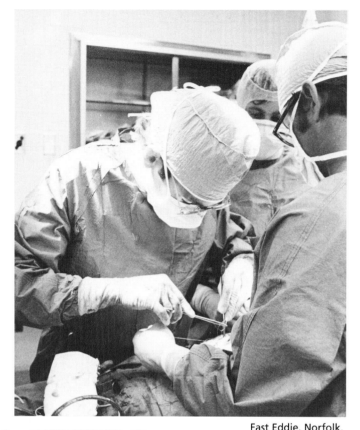

Fast Eddie, Norfolk,
Virginia, 1977

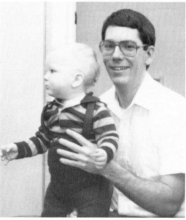

Jonathan Edward,
#1 Son, 1983

I can see your
tonsils, Dad!

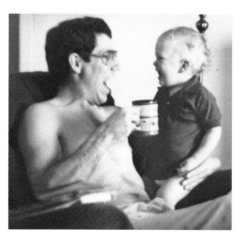

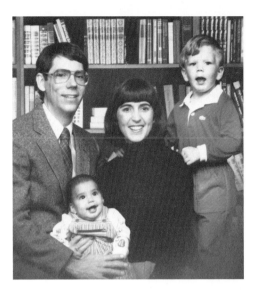

David Michael
joins the family,
1985

Storytime

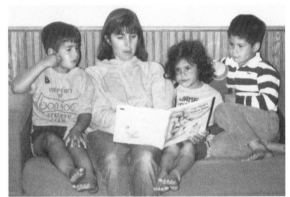

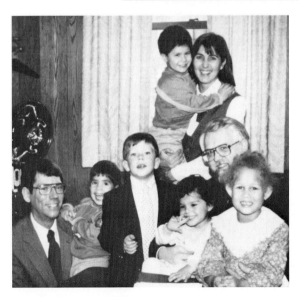

Judge Larry
Starcher finalizes
adoption papers
for Victoria,
Jonathan Wayne,
and Christina,
November 1988

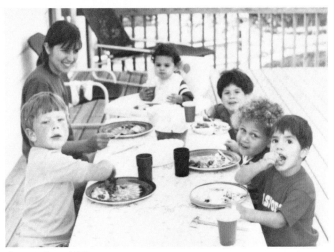

Suppertime, 1987

1983

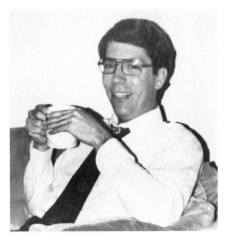

Time to move
the firewood,
late fall, 1988

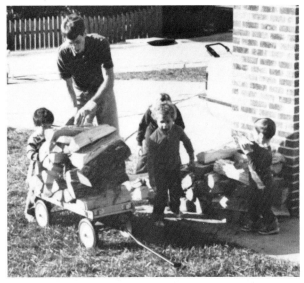

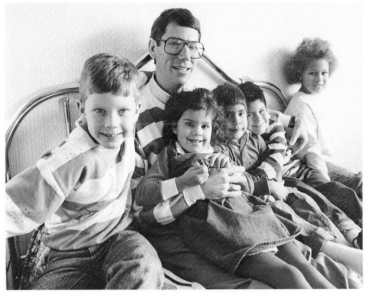

Valley Forge, Pennsylvania, November 1990

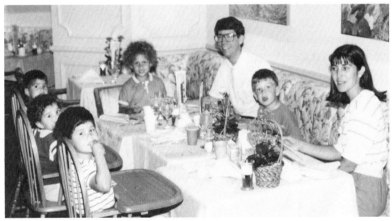

November 1988 Weekend trip to Pittsburgh.

Ed discusses writing a book with David Biebel

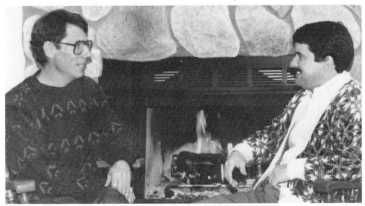

David Biebel

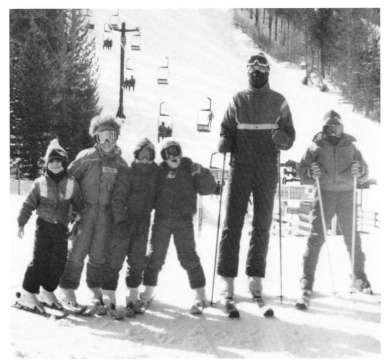

Winter 1992 vacation at Ski Brule, Michigan

Lake Michigan beach on way to Detroit, 1989

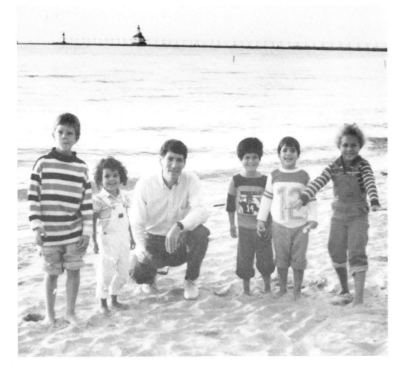

9

Everything You Wanted
to Know—
And Were Not Afraid to Ask

*e*verywhere we go, people from reporters to lay-
men to young people, ask lots of questions about
AIDS. Since we can't devote a chapter to each
concern, perhaps the best approach is to choose
some of the most common ones and give you a brief
response.

**1. What's the difference between HIV-infection and
AIDS—and which do you have?**

AIDS (**A**cquired **I**mmuno**D**eficiency **S**yndrome) is the
end stage of infection with HIV (**H**uman **I**mmunodeficiency
Virus). In other words, HIV is the AIDS virus. It gradually
disables a person's immune system until infectious agents
such as bacteria, fungi, other viruses, parasites, and some
cancers are able to cause illness or even death. In a healthy

97

person, these intruders would be recognized and destroyed by the body's natural defenses.

Because HIV works slowly, the symptoms of AIDS often develop over a long period of time. For years there was an intermediate classification: ARC (**A**IDS **R**elated **C**omplex) to describe HIV-positive patients with certain symptoms but not full-blown AIDS. In early 1992, the CDC proposed that anyone whose T4-cell count fell below 200 (from a normal 1,000) should be classified as a person with AIDS.

According to this new classification, when my HIV status became known in 1989, I already had AIDS, even though I had no obvious AIDS symptoms. Over the next two years, my T4-cell count fell to nearly zero without my developing the more severe manifestations of the syndrome (group of symptoms) known as AIDS.

2. How close are we to finding a vaccine or cure?

I have met Dr. Bob Redfield of Walter Reed, who published an article in the New England Journal of Medicine (June 1991) about how work is proceeding on a vaccine that seems to have some promise. But there are many problems to overcome, so I think it will be years rather than months before a vaccine is perfected, if it ever happens.

This is a tricky virus, not like the one that causes polio. HIV changes; it becomes resistant. And once it's in the body, it gets incorporated into the patient's molecular structure and then reproduces itself. It is nearly impossible to isolate and destroy without killing the patient in the process. The only "cure" I can imagine at this point would be through divine healing.

3. Have you met people whom the Lord has physically healed of AIDS?

Not personally, although we're beginning to hear accounts. For instance, a 1991 issue of *Charisma* magazine included the testimony of a young man who was healed. Certainly God's will is to do this, since he is more powerful than any disease process. In fact, I have received my healing. This happened not because I'm some special person who deserves it more than others, but because of who God is. (See chapter 12.) The Word of God is very clear on the issue of healing. If Jesus could raise Lazarus from the dead, in effect reversing all the processes of decay that three days in the grave would bring about, routing out HIV from my system would be mild by comparison. It matters not to me how he does it, whether by miracle or by medicine, for all healing is in his hands. More than just physical, healing involves the soul and the spirit. The amazing fact is that the Lord provides strength during these times.

4. As a Christian physician, what are some of your thoughts about Magic Johnson's disclosure in late 1991?

You don't have to be a Christian to be disappointed with his initial press conference. I think he started speaking before he himself was educated about "safe sex." Furthermore, Magic downplayed any reference to abstinence, so for President Bush to call him a hero tended to cloud the issue. I'm glad he came forward with his diagnosis, but he lost an important opportunity to educate millions of fans, especially young people, about the dangers (and immorality) of sexual promiscuity.

Right after that, I accepted an invitation from a local school nurse who said, "Ed, can you come down? Kids are coming in saying safe sex is okay." I put it to them straight, you can count on that. You should have seen their faces when I rolled up my sleeve and showed them the HIV-related shingles I had at the time. "You don't want to get this," I assured them, "or any of the other much worse problems that go with HIV infection. And you don't have to, either. If you'll just save sex until marriage, and remain faithful to an uninfected spouse, there is almost no chance that you'll get it."

5. What is the risk of patients' acquiring HIV from health-care workers?

So far, there are very few documented cases of patients who became infected from exposure to infected health professionals. The chance may be only one in a million—but nobody really knows for sure. This is because an exchange of body fluids must occur to transfer the virus, and the only way this happens is in some type of accident during an invasive procedure.

In reality, health-care workers are more at risk of becoming infected from their patients than the other way around. So I favor testing patients prior to invasive procedures, when possible, and certainly when they admit to engaging in high-risk behavior. (Of course, patients are not always truthful about that.) It's always better to know these facts before beginning treatment—and to prevent transmission to others.

6. Should there be premarital testing for HIV?

That depends on what kind of behavior patterns the prospective bride and groom have had and whether they are willing to be truthful. (Rent or buy the video "No Second Chance" from Jeremiah films to see the intergenerational agony one family endured because of this.) People who are getting married should have a physical, at which time they can discuss HIV testing with their doctor. The safest course is for anybody who has ever been sexually active with *anyone* but the intended spouse to be tested. At stake is the health of both the marital partner and any children who result from the union.

7. Why haven't the American Medical Association (AMA) and other medical groups done more to protect their members and the public?

I am not a member of the AMA. (I dropped my mem bership because of their pro-abortion stance.) Normally they endorse CDC guidelines, but when the testing proposals came out, there was a lot of resistance. Regardless of how loudly some medical professionals protest that the risk to patients is less than this or that, I believe that what really drives them is the desire for autonomy and self-preservation (otherwise known as greed). However, I am encouraged that the AMA has moved in a more responsible direction toward HIV testing.

The American people are driving this issue now! Some call it public "hysteria" but at least the once-silent majority is finally being heard. HIV is not a disease like syphilis or gonorrhea, which is usually cured by an injection in the hip. It is subtle and diabolical in the way it spreads, because the majority of people who are HIV-infected don't know they have it. There are probably at least a million cases in this country alone, and some say that is a very conservative estimate! Only ASAP has been outspoken about efforts to protect the public from this epidemic.

8. Aren't you angry that you got an HIV infection from a patient?

You might get a different answer from Donna, but I've never held it against whoever it was. That patient probably didn't even know he or she had it. (In 1985 we were just starting to test for HIV.) I've even talked with Jonathan Edward about this, because I thought when he got older he might develop a deep resentment toward all homosexuals and drug addicts, groups within which AIDS has been most prevalent. However, if anyone is to blame, it is members of the medical establishment who dragged their feet in terms of keeping health professionals informed.

9. Do you favor mandatory testing for health-care workers and patients?

I favor mandatory testing on a periodic basis depending on geographical assessment of risk factors. For example, when a recent patient sample was done of emergency-room patients in a northeastern city, 7 percent were found to be HIV-positive. If that number were coming in with cancer, strokes, or the like, we would be moving heaven and earth to find out what was causing it and how the cause could be controlled. But if patients come in with HIV, we just send them back out, thinking "Isn't that awful?" Therefore if a health-care worker is in a high-incidence area, he or she should be tested frequently.

Not long after my visit to the CDC, the American College of Surgeons came out against the guidelines. I believe that physicians should regard their profession as a sacred trust on behalf of their patients. We owe it to our patients to have regular medical care ourselves, especially if we are HIV-positive, so that someone else can be sure our judgment is not clouded. We need checks and balances in regard to HIV, just as we have with physicians who have problems with drugs and alcohol.

In some health-care settings, such as general medicine and nursing, there are many noninvasive procedures performed for which retraining may not be necessary. However, health-care workers with HIV will fall through the net, unable to find something else to do. That's where details like disability insurance and workmen's compensation have to be worked out. It's going to cost money, but that is no reason to keep us from doing what is right.

I say to my fellow surgeons that it is illogical not to want to know your HIV status, for your own good as well as the good of your patients. "First of all, do no harm." Most of us dislike having nonprofessionals tell us what to do. I know that, and so do you. But shouldn't we do this on our own? Testing has to do with knowledge versus ignorance. To provide the best treatment, we need to know everything we can about a particular patient—family history, what medications are being taken, past diseases and surgeries. All that information is important, as is knowing a patient's HIV status—and our own.

10. Aren't people afraid of what might happen if the test shows them to be HIV-positive?

That is a very poor argument against testing! Wouldn't you want to find out if you are infected, so you can get early treatment and take precautions against getting certain types of opportunistic diseases? You can also be careful not to transmit it to other people. Surely you would want to have this information and use it in the best interest of others and yourself.

It's pretty simple, really, but the other side comes on very strong with some inane reasoning: "We can't afford it." Or "It violates my privacy." And so on. I say that the fear of diagnosis must never override the need to know. Good, sound medicine is based on facts, not emotions.

11. What do you think the general public really wants here?

People want to be confident they're not going to be exposed to this disease through a health-care worker. I think they deserve that consideration. Although the risk can never be reduced to zero, they want to see that something has been done to make it as low as possible. So far, they don't see it being done.

The public is waking up to how the agenda for AIDS has been politicized and manipulated by various special-interest groups. As a result, the real threat of the disease has been kept hidden. For example, some homosexual activists have resisted the idea of testing because it "violates civil rights" or is "an invasion of privacy." Others cite discrimination against homosexuals as the reason there has been inadequate funding of AIDS research and treatment programs. On the other hand, at first some public health officials were saying there was little chance for a patient to transmit the virus to a health-care worker (and vice versa). They knew it could happen at the time, though they said something different. They also lied by implying that AIDS was a problem only for homosexuals and IV drug abusers.

So the public says, "Whoa, you lied to us. Now we don't believe anything you say." It is going to take a while to regain public confidence. I think the CDC is on the right track, but, unfortunately, they don't have the cooperation of some of the medical groups.

12. But isn't AIDS still really a homosexual disease?

AIDS can no longer be viewed as a threat to only such "high risk" groups as homosexuals and IV drug users. It is *everyone's* problem now, as my own case has proven! Not only are health-care workers its potential victims, but HIV is being found in increasing numbers among heterosexuals, as well as in babies born to infected mothers. Nevertheless, some people (especially conservative evangelicals) seem to think, "We can stop this plague right now by dealing with the sinners who caused it!" As if it's not *our* problem, and the way to stop it is to do something about "them." Well— and I want to emphasize this clearly—nothing is going to completely halt HIV's gradually increasing death-grip on humanity until the Lord returns. But there's a lot we can do to control its spread.

I'm thinking globally here, not provincially, like many North American Christians often do when they consider

HIV disease, as well as other things. Even if someday a vaccine or cure becomes available here, it will almost certainly not be readily available in the Third World, where AIDS will continue to march on.

It is also very presumptuous—and *untrue*—to say that HIV only happens to "bad people." Morality alone does not guarantee immunity to this or any other disease so long as we live in an imperfect world.

Worldwide, believers and nonbelievers alike are suffering (and will suffer) because of AIDS. Regardless of how these patients acquired the disease, it is simply not right to turn our backs on them and their families as if they brought the plague on themselves. If I read the Bible correctly, we are *all* sinners and under God's judgment. And people are going to keep sinning until the final coming of God's kingdom. However, for the Christian the penalty has been paid by Jesus.

If God can include an adulterer and murderer like King David in the very lineage of Jesus the Redeemer, we ought to pause and look in the mirror of our own consciences before we write off those "bad people."

13. If abstinence and/or marital fidelity—not "safe sex"—is the answer, why don't more doctors preach it?

I hate to be this blunt, but I think it's mainly because they are reluctant to deal with their own immorality. Having grown up in an era of sexual freedom, they don't want to restrict their own activities—and it's pretty difficult to convince others of something if you really don't believe it yourself. As far as I'm concerned, you can apply this same thought to politicians, preachers, and other public figures who resist proclaiming the surest way to keep AIDS from spreading: abstinence before marriage and faithfulness within marriage.

14. Should Christian medical personnel treat AIDS patients, even if it means risking their lives?

That's a difficult question with a simple answer—yes. Jumping into a raging stream to save somebody is about as risky as treating somebody with HIV disease. Yet, especially if you are a Christian, you wouldn't think twice about jumping into that stream, even though you know there's a potential to lose your own life in the process.

Christian health-care workers ought to be leaders in this role. I met a dentist who actually recruits AIDS patients, though in a quiet way so he doesn't scare off his other patients. He sees that as a ministry, and that's the attitude we all should take. Not everyone will want to work only with AIDS patients, but I think we Christians ought to be leading the way by showing our compassion, and not by words alone. I don't mean Christians should be reckless in any way. God gave us a brain to process facts and use them wisely. In this case, that means taking proper precautions.

15. I'm a Christian health-care worker who believes that God has called me to minister to AIDS patients, even at risk to myself. But aren't there family issues involved?

I think we've rarely had issues of this magnitude brought before us, although Christians have always been willing to minister to victims of hepatitis, leprosy, tuberculosis, and the plague. Of course, some physicians ran and refused to get involved with these and certain other communicable diseases. I can't answer for them.

This is a highly personal issue that depends a great deal on spiritual maturity. Because the transmission risk is never zero where HIV is concerned, it should also be a decision agreeable to your spouse. Doing invasive procedures on HIV patients, whether in surgery or nursing, will involve some risk. If your spouse agrees that the risk is worth taking to have a ministry to those patients, I believe you should accept God's call and use your medical skills on their behalf.

16. Where do precautions end and risks begin, and how does faith in God blur that line?

Take the setting of a missionary health provider who doesn't have access to double-gloving (maybe there are no gloves at all or none without holes), or who has to reuse needles that cannot be properly sterilized. In that case, you completely rely on the Lord. I've been in situations where needles must be used hundreds of times. Or scalpels are so dull, you have to put your whole weight on them to make them cut through the skin. Yet they can't be resharpened. Because gloves must sometimes be reused and repowdered, you never really know what their status is.

But those things don't seem to be that important if it is clear that God called you there. So you rely on his power and protection. I don't mean that you jump into the raging stream without knowing how to swim, for we should never "test" God. We just have to be in the Word, confessing and believing it, and then go about the work he puts before us. When I was on the mission field, it never dawned on me to be concerned about catching a disease—and I never did.

17. Do people look at you differently than they did before?

I suppose some people look at me and think, What a shame. How do you do it? You used to be a cardiac surgeon and now you have to deal with this. My answer would be that being a cardiac surgeon is great stuff, but it's not the whole world. It's not even the top of anything. The top depends on what God wants you to do. As far as I'm concerned, the guy who cleans the church is just as important as I.

One problem with cardiac surgery is that you sort of get pushed there up a long, tough road. You really pay your dues, so you enjoy the fact that people look up to you. It's hard not to believe you've earned their respect and deserve it.

My way of validating that respect was to try to always do the best I could for my patients. I never considered myself any better than anybody else, though I enjoyed very much what I did, as well as the benefits. You have to guard yourself against pride whether you're a surgeon or a preacher, or maybe even a very good janitor.

Although I would much rather still be operating, God has given me an opportunity to do something else, medically and in other ways. I want to be an example to HIV-infected health-care workers and anyone else who is impacted by this disease, showing them that even in the face of AIDS, life goes on. In fact, impossible though it may seem, in spite of HIV infection, or perhaps because of it, life can be better than it ever was before. If this revelation encourages one person to come into the kingdom of God, then the process will have validity for me.

△ **10** ▷

Becoming a Soul Doctor

n the world's history of plagues, AIDS could end up being the worst ever, and not just in a physical sense. It has the stigma of *leprosy*, the transmission characteristics of *syphilis*, the natural history of *tuberculosis* and the prognosis (at least so far) of *the bubonic plague*. Additionally, its long-term global socioeconomic impact may be greater than all the wars ever fought.

In times of plague, responses to its victims have ranged from desertion to persecution to compassion. In the Middle Ages, many physicians and clergy fled the cities during a plague. For example, in London's plague of 1665, when nearly 70,000 died, only 13 doctors stayed to care for the 200,000 citizens who were left in the city. Modern people with HIV infection have experienced similar abandonment.

Persecution and scapegoating is society's second most common response to plagues. In Milan, Italy, in 1630, two men—a barber-surgeon and the commissioner of health—were accused of spreading disease by means of deadly ointments. The city senate ordered that their flesh should be torn with red-hot pincers, their right hands cut off, their bones broken, and that they should then be put on a torture wheel for six hours before being burned at the stake.

In the late twentieth century, HIV-infected people are persecuted more subtly but no less unfairly. They may have their employment and health benefits cut off instead of their hands. To my knowledge, none have been burned at the stake, but in Florida one family's house was destroyed by arson. Nobody needs to put HIV-infected people on the wheel. They're already being tortured enough.

Persecution and abandonment have always been ways to disenfranchise the poor and the plague-prone. The net result is a fragmented and demoralized society in which any epidemic will continue to spread. Sound familiar? How else can we understand—more than a decade into this plague's history—our nation's continuing failure to develop a rational approach to AIDS, a multifaceted (political, public health/medical, educational, and ecclesiastical) policy and agenda? Compassion is the only helpful response to those afflicted by a plague, and the only one we should allow. Physician William Boghurst remained in London to care for patients during one severe plague. His conviction was that professionals must accept the responsibilities as well as the benefits. Ministers must preach, captains must fight, physicians must attend to the sick.

When HIV-infected people are treated with compassion, not only do *they* benefit, but those who help them are rewarded in less tangible ways (active love always receives more than it gives). As this happens, societal disruption is inhibited and even reversed, because hysteria cannot be maintained in the midst of composed, courageous people who are calmly caring for the afflicted.

Besides these practical arguments for compassion, we who claim to be followers of Jesus of Nazareth have in him the example of someone who touched the lepers and ministered to all the disenfranchised of his society. To him, their needs were not a burden; they were an opportunity to bring God's comfort, grace, and presence into the life context of people who knew nothing but despair.

I know it is difficult to think of AIDS as anything other than a threat, a crisis you may be living with already, or one that is lurking on the horizon. But did you know that in some Eastern languages the word *crisis* combines the root words for "danger" and "opportunity"? AIDS is obviously a danger, but might it also be an opportunity in disguise? It has been for me, and I'm convinced it can be for you, too, whether or not you are HIV-positive.

In the final few chapters of this book, I want to examine four facets of this one theme—"AIDS as an opportunity"—without discounting the fact that for me, for you, for our society, and for the world it is also a dangerous crisis of monstrous proportions.

Because I want to reserve my most personal thoughts until last, we will look first at AIDS as an opportunity for both health professionals and others, especially those within the church. Then I'll share some rather painfully gained insights about HIV-infected persons and their families. After that, I'll take you behind closed doors into my own family and marriage, concluding with an even closer look at the one component of this whole danger/opportunity that has kept me from going over the edge in a personal sense.

In terms of health-care workers, including physicians, compassion is increasing, but it has been a slow process and there is still a long way to go. By compassion, I mean more than sensitivity in terms of individual patient needs—and AIDS patients usually take more time and energy than those with other diseases. Even more basic is the humane choice to treat HIV-infected people rather than referring them elsewhere.

At the risk of being labeled "homophobic" (a meaningless term), I think the militant behavior of the homosexual community has worked against its own best interests and the rest of us in the area of AIDS-related concerns. I cannot fathom how they can believe that the way to engender compassion for HIV-infected people is by disrupting public gatherings, abusing elected officials, holding noisy parades, and carrying belligerent placards.

This combative activity confuses rather than clarifies the issues of AIDS patients, many of whom are not homosexuals.

Compassion and the Health-Care Professional

I would choose medicine again as a profession if I had it all to do over, especially if I could know at the start what I never learned about illness before becoming HIV-positive. Of course, I wish I had known more about AIDS when I was retrained, so I could have been more careful. Because nothing was said about it to us residents, I just went on my merry way.

Perhaps AIDS is one reason there is a nursing shortage and fewer qualified people applying to medical school these days. But, as far as I'm concerned, becoming a health professional is still one of the most fulfilling callings. The key word there is "calling." In the age of AIDS, you may not make it if you enter health-care work in search of wealth or power, or even because in a purely human sense you care about people and want to help them. You will eventually become cynical, burned out, or both—unless you truly feel *called* to be a caregiver.

When I talk to Christian medical groups, I often ask a simple question: "Do you have an upward calling from God? If so, what is it?" One of the rewards of following Jesus Christ is becoming convinced that your profession is a divine calling. This is the key to understanding what kept the apostle Paul going in spite of the discouragements and hardships of trying to carry Christianity to a pagan world. How else can we explain his joy and contentment, even when imprisoned?

If you are a Christian who has chosen a health-related career, are you just working like the rest of the world, as if the opportunity to minister through medicine is merely a job, a way to earn a living? That's the way it was for me once, although I did try to take a personal interest in my patients. Before HIV rearranged my life in so many ways, I seldom stopped to ask myself, "What am I really doing here?" I was cruising along, enjoying the ride and even deeply grateful for God's providence and grace. But I had blinders on. I was so focused on repairing people's hearts that I often missed the equally if not more significant opportunity to minister to their deeper needs, to help repair their souls and spirits. I cringe to think of the eternal consequences of this omission, especially for those who died during surgery. I was trained as a technician, a specialist in body repair, and that was my main concern.

To minister effectively to HIV-infected individuals as a medical professional, you must ask yourself this question: *"What am I trying to accomplish through my relationship with this patient?"* The disease model you learned in your training will eventually prove inadequate in the face of the frustrating, long-term, irreversible decline you will see in many of these patients. If you think that your only role is to cure disease, AIDS will have you for lunch. You will quickly begin looking for somebody you can really cure, rationalizing that "I should be a more productive steward of my hi-tech training and skills."

Interestingly enough, that same frustration's other side is where the real opportunity for ministry through medicine begins. But, to pursue it, you have to view a patient wholistically: body/soul/spirit, existing in a web of horizontal and vertical relationships constantly in need of maintenance and repair. Sometimes there is *nothing* you can do physically, beyond trying to make your patient more comfortable—and the medical treatment you offer may have just the opposite effect. But you can *always* be a "soul doctor," if only through a simple prayer, reading an encouraging Bible passage, or just sitting with him or her silently for a while, a partner on the pilgrimage of pain.

One opportunity AIDS gave me was to learn firsthand that pain has many faces. It might be the pain of hearing the ear-nose-throat specialist's trocar needle crunching through the cartilage of my nose because he needed to culture the bugs causing a year-long sinus infection that the antibiotics hadn't touched. Or it might have been the pain of not being able to do things I used to do and the feeling that now my life was useless.

Having to strip down and put on a gown for an upper-gastrointestinal and gallbladder ultrasound brings its own kind of pain. Or being ignored, even ostracized by your friends. Or wondering if you should go swimming in the public pool with your kids, or hug and kiss them like you used to. Or wondering how much your illness is going to drain your family's physical, emotional, and financial reserves before it's all over. There is also self-pity, confusion, loneliness, emptiness, doubt, fear, and the sense of isolation that is a side effect of feeling abandoned by others as well as God.

Pain is pain, and even when there's no pill, surgery, or cure available, health professionals can always help in some way if they fight the temptation to withdraw when there's nothing more that can be done medically. I know you have too much to do, and many other patients—some of whom God may even cure through your efforts. However, beyond the thoughts of failure and inconvenience lies a seldom-charted territory of discovery—for you and your patient, especially if he or she is a believer. There is no doubt in my mind that as people get nearer to death (or even think they are), if they can get past all the negative stuff that can go with dying, they begin to see realities much more clearly. The jewels of wisdom they have to offer could never be found by search or study—only by being there and listening.

Some dying patients have a vision of heaven or angels, or even of the Lord himself, and will share it with you. I urge you to accept these experiences as special gifts. How else could you know such things, except by lying there yourself? Through your patient's situation, you may be blessed and touched by a deep sense of the reality and presence of the Divine. Treasure such gifts forever, for they are priceless.

Sometimes there may be only abject suffering, over-whelming and apparently meaningless. Even then, by choosing to enter into that pain, you will diminish your patient's hurt and sorrow. And you will be blessed as you struggle to understand, for any believer who embraces this search with an open mind will inevitably end up gazing at the cross, where the guiltless Redeemer cried out, "My God, my God, why have you forsaken me?"

The Church and Its AIDS Ministry

In the midst of all the mental groping and grappling that comes to any health-care worker, those who are Christians should also see this disease as an opportunity to lead, convict, convince, inspire, and educate the church about the need for other believers to take on this ministry. Of all institutions, the church is the only one designed by God to be a caring community, representing him in a tangible way in a world that has always been hurting. Why else would the church be called the body of Christ? Surely it is God's intention that we who claim allegiance to him carry his unchanging love to the very people sought out by his Son during his earthly sojourn.

As far as I can tell, the conservative branches of the North American church have failed so far to minister adequately to HIV-infected persons, *for several unacceptable reasons.* In the early days of AIDS, probably because the disease was perceived as a homosexual problem, the evangelical perspective was generally more judgmental than it is today. One of the reasons this self-righteous attitude is changing is illustrated by the story of a conservative pastor's daughter who became infected through her boyfriend at a time when the policy of her father's church was to have nothing to do with "the sinners" who contracted AIDS. Only the most sanctimonious would dare bar his own flesh and blood from the very help she would desperately need in the next few years.

Unfortunately, the more typical story thus far has been like that of one young pastor and his family. His wife was infected with HIV through a 1985 blood transfusion during the birth of their first child. Subsequently, she gave birth to another child, who was born with AIDS, although some babies born to infected mothers remain uninfected. This pastor first became a bereaved father, as the child slowly succumbed to the disease. Next, the church he was serving asked him to leave. Soon after that, he became a widower.

The point here is that AIDS is coming to your town, to your schools, to your church and maybe even to your family. This is no longer debatable. Because it's *our* problem already, the question is not: "If it comes to us, what shall our *policy* be?" The proper question for the church to be asking is framed in terms of human need, not theological principles: "How can we touch the lives of people with AIDS and their families in the name of Jesus Christ?"

To do this effectively, there are at least three more bridges to cross after a church acknowledges its responsibility for an AIDS ministry. These are credibility, sensitivity, and capability. Setting up programs and hiring people to represent the congregation is not enough, even if it is a start. One reason some churches are so ineffective today is that many laypeople think that "ministry" is what they pay their pastors to do, instead of what their pastors should be equipping *them* to do.

The only way to bridge the credibility gap is for as many members as possible to get personally involved in a ministry to AIDS patients. I'm not talking about the "politics" of AIDS here. Some Christians think they've gotten "involved" by writing letters or making phone calls, or maybe even providing financial support. But you cannot really understand this illness by staying at a safe distance and shooting arrows, thinking you're doing the "right" thing. Jesus said ". . . whatever you did for one of the least of these brothers of mine, you did for me" (Matt. 25:40 NIV). The *right* thing is to get down and get dirty. Until you've done that, despite how sympathetically you speak about HIV-infected people, your words are meaningless, and people listening will say, "What do you really know about it?"

Sensitivity, like credibility, is not something you can manufacture, either. It means knowing someone's specific needs and caring about that person. So you have to do more listening than talking, a difficult challenge for any Christian who is used to handing out advice laced with pious platitudes and Bible verses. AIDS patients may need and want *some* of that, but sensitivity means sharing your faith gifts on their turf, according to their timing, and at their request.

If listening is difficult for some lay Christians, it is doubly difficult for the clergy, who are so used to holding forth in situations they control, such as in church or at a funeral or even in visitation. Few of them are very prepared for a cardiac surgeon to walk unannounced into their office one dark day in May and say, "I really need to talk to somebody, pastor. A few weeks ago I learned I'm infected with the AIDS virus, and my life feels like it's been turned upside down."

When I said that, my former pastor just sat there with his mouth open, totally shocked for a few moments. Then he said, "I don't know what to say." That's not a bad place to start, because there may be nothing you *can* say that will fix things. But, if you start like that, you might add ". . . but I love you, and we'll do everything we can to help." Then you might say, "I've read some and thought a lot about this disease, but would you help me better understand what it means personally? Please, tell me everything you've been experiencing, and how I can help."

Anyone who wants to minister in the name of Jesus to people infected with HIV needs first to go before God and examine his or her attitudes toward AIDS, toward the patient, even toward death itself. I'm not talking about numbered prayer arrows you aim at God to tell him this or that or ask him for such and such. What you will need is wrestling, agonizing prayer, because getting involved with AIDS will chew you up and spit you out if you are not ministering in the power of the Holy Spirit. If you ask, "Lord, show me how to deal with the problem of AIDS," you will never help anybody. But if you ask, "Lord, show me ways to really help people with AIDS," you are headed in the right direction. Ask God to act through you. Take into your heart and put into action the realization that Christians "abide in Him and He in us, because He has given us of His Spirit" (1 John 4:13).

Sometimes the first response to an HIV-infected person is to reach for the pastoral-care Rolodex, with its list of problems and solutions. But AIDS is too complicated for an A-B-C approach. It is neither appropriate nor helpful to reel off such simplistic answers as "All you have to do is pray. Then follow these five steps [or go through these three stages] and everything will be hunky-dory."

An effective AIDS ministry involves *everybody:* the patients, their families, the church at large, and its clergy. "Why?" questions abound, but nobody can really answer them. So the only helpful answers are relational and personal: "I care about you and hurt with you, brother [sister]. You're not going to face this alone, because I'm here, and I'll be here until you don't need me anymore."

Now, that's light-years more helpful than stopping by just long enough to say, "Call me if you need me!"—with the last word hanging in the air as you turn to go. You can bet the farm the patient is not going to call, even if he has one foot in the grave, because he knows what you would say: "Sorry, I can't come right now, but be sure to call again." But what are some practical ways to help? Why not begin by looking for a need you can meet and then just do it? For example, the gutters on our house needed cleaning and in my condition there was no way I could get up there. So one day our sixty-year-old interim pastor showed up and said, "I'm going to clean your gutters." And he climbed up on a ladder in the rain and cold and did the ones he could reach. One of the deacons came over after that and cleaned the second-story gutters, also without our asking.

That's the kind of help AIDS patients need. Take them a meal you've prepared, something that can be frozen in case they don't need it right then. While you're there, discreetly observe other things that aren't getting done, either because that person hasn't the strength or is so depressed he can't get motivated. For instance, offer to do the laundry or the cleaning, or to repair something that may not be working quite right. Ask if a ride somewhere is needed, or if you can do some shopping or pick up some medication. Invite him or her to go on a picnic with your family, or maybe to a ball game or concert. Things like this speak volumes, while pious platitudes with no real feelings to support them are just so much sound and fury, signifying nothing—except to you.

Ask yourself, "What would I be willing to do for this person if he were my brother or sister? Genuine kindness has as its root the idea of being of the same kind: "kindred." If you can reach the point of treating an infected person as a relative, you've come a long way. In fact, like the good Samaritan in Jesus' parable, you demonstrate the meaning of "love your neighbor as yourself" whenever you show kindness to a wounded traveler on the road of life.

One other thing: If you really want to show that you care, how about a hug? This disease has such power to isolate infected people from their families and friends. They will feel reconnected with the living, instead of the dying, if somebody reaches out to them in that way.

That's the way it felt to me when I started going to a different church. Believers' Church and World Outreach Center in Marshfield provided me with a living gospel that nourished me both spiritually and physically. The pastor and congregation welcomed me with hugs, acceptance, and expectation. I described this feeling in one of the few poems I have ever written:

The Hug
God drew me here,
this World Outreach Center.
At first, a Handshake, a Hello.
Then laying on of hands.
Next,
A Hug: Brother, let's sit down and talk.
How are you dealing with this?
Late night discussion by way of modem?
Does the Holy Spirit traverse electronic wires?
The appointment: another Hug
But I have AIDS!
Hang on, Revelation's coming!
God wants me healed!
Listening, Praise, Encouragement, Prayer and a Hug.
Family!
This is His plan:
"Thy Kingdom come, on earth as it is in Heaven."

⊿11⊳

Letting Your Love Grow

Studies have shown that people with terminal diseases are most afraid of two things: that they will die in great pain or that they may die alone.

Medication is no guarantee that an HIV-infected person will not die in pain—short of narcotizing the patient into oblivion. There are so many variations of end-stage AIDS that nobody can be sure how it will be until that time arrives. However, the family and friends of a patient can alleviate the second fear by making this commitment and keeping it: "We are with you in this and will be until it's over." Faithfulness like this provides the context for love to grow, even if it has not been there very much in the past.

On the other hand, love's growth is stifled if an infected person just withdraws or sits back and waits for help to come. He must reach out to people, let them inside his thoughts and feelings. Sometimes, patients will have to minister to others, giving out even when their own tank is empty. We who are infected may have to help *others* think positively, giving *them* hope, even when we ourselves may be

121

sliding toward the edge of despair. Real love grows in two directions.

"Dear Patient . . ."

First things first: HIV-infected people have to be realistic. Once you know you're HIV-positive, you can't just go about your business as if nothing has happened. It's a new chapter in your life. Ignoring it or denying it will not help. You first need to find a physician you can trust, somebody you can call when the office is closed. This should be someone who will level with you about the twists and turns that lie ahead of you, and will covenant with you (an old concept, but the basis of good medicine) to go there as your fellow traveler.

Another aspect of that "realistic" approach is acknowledging that your lifestyle will change, in terms of nutrition, for instance. There may be activities you'll no longer be able to do, and medications with unpleasant side effects. For me, accepting new limitations has been very difficult, maybe because there never seemed to be anything I couldn't do if I put my mind to it. Times have changed! For instance, once I was taking a shower when my blood count was so far down that my blood pressure plunged and I had to stagger to bed and lie down quickly before I fainted. There have been many times I was sick from AZT to the point of not being able to eat, although I desperately wanted to regain those pounds (I lost twenty pounds originally and ten more with chemo) I had lost since 1985. Even relatively "minor" things like the chronic sinus infection I had for more than a year (despite four rounds of antibiotics) really wore me down. Besides putting up with all the yucky stuff that kept coming out of my nose, the inability of my system to dispatch such a simple bug was another frustration and a less-than-subtle reminder that I was infected. That got old pretty fast for a guy who was used to being healthy as a horse.

The list goes on. There was a pesky eye infection that would sometimes be bad enough that I couldn't see very well. The idea of going blind is frightening to anyone, but the eye infection also kept me from reading what had kept my head above water, the Bible. I remember praying, "You know, Lord, if something happens to my eyes, I've got tapes of the Bible to listen to. I'm ready."

But the worst things I faced giving up were activities I wanted to do with the kids, such as hunting and fishing. I wondered if I should risk getting so far out in the woods that I might not be able to make it back. Once when I took the kids fishing on the farm in southern Georgia, just walking down to the lake nearly killed me, and I wondered, "Should I be doing this?"

AIDS changes the way you look at everything! Yet hidden in all this upheaval and change was the opportunity to see life and its meaning with more clarity. For instance, I used to be as compulsive at home as I was in surgery. The precision needed in my work carried over into the home as an insistence that there is a right way to do things, to schedule activities, to keep the house, and so on. Sometimes I treated the kids and Donna as if I were a king, and they were my subjects. (I am not happy or proud about telling you this.)

I always had a list of projects, especially things needing repairs. It was a never-ending list, because as soon as we fixed one thing, another would get broken. Five kids and a dog will take care of that! Even after I got sick, I maintained my list, so there was always a vague anxiety that if I wasn't fixing something, I hadn't looked hard enough. You can imagine the kind of conflict I brought into our home, now that I had hours available every day, instead of saving up my projects for the weekends. To get beyond that, I had to realize that some of those things I was so focused on wouldn't matter a lick in five years, maybe even in one year.

Realism, however, doesn't mean being fatalistic about *everything*. Whether sick or well, all of us must learn to be realistic about things that are actually important. Sort these out, using the new discernment that becoming an HIV-infected patient can provide. Then you'll begin to appreciate the basic things you took for granted before: health, freedom, love, life itself.

To do this, you'll have to deal with the intense loneliness and fear that AIDS brings. Its propensity to isolate—even to the point of isolating you from the real "you"—will have to be faced. Otherwise, you'll give in to feeling like a leper and allow an invisible wall to be built between others and yourself.

The underlying problem is that someone who hasn't been there can never really understand our situation. We who are infected with HIV need to tell others how we feel, and that takes more energy than we think we have. But the investment will be worth making in the long run, because it may help heal the hurt that those who really care about us carry as they participate with us in whatever bad things AIDS is doing to us at the moment.

I have been on both sides, as observer and patient, and I believe it's almost as hard to suffer with somebody you love as it is for the patient himself or herself. One thing's for sure, though. You'll do a lot better with this if you prepare yourself for it. The fact is, people react differently, even to the same pain or loss.

Both sides have the option of withdrawing, and with AIDS the temptation to do so is very strong. As family members look into the future and see only pain and separation, the natural thing to do is to protect themselves by withdrawing, at least emotionally if not physically. I've seen this happen, even in the health-care setting. Here's a patient with HIV in the bed; a doctor walks in and stands way over there, and a nurse comes in and stands in the far corner. If they do get any closer, you get the feeling they are hiding behind an invisible shield. Observing this withdrawal is nothing like having it done to you, I promise you. This common reaction does not mean that health-care workers are afraid of contracting HIV from a patient. Rather, it is a result of dealing with their fears about what is to come.

We who are infected with HIV need to gently invite our caregivers to find a way to bypass that emotional wall. They may be struggling not only with a sense of impending failure to help us, and the guilt that goes with that, but also with the practicalities of dealing with our infections, cancers, GI problems, central IV lines, or feeding tubes. The reality is that the whole scenario with respect to the physical problems can become almost intolerable for a caregiver.

Because of our illness, the people caring for us must daily enter the distressing world of our loneliness, confusion, debility, pain, and a multitude of weird things that a compassionate mind would hope could never happen to the human body. Is it any wonder they sometimes feel ambivalence, an approach-avoidance conflict of enormous proportions? They care, but they hurt, too.

Perhaps it seems easier to just get mad at them, to feel so sorry for ourselves that we withdraw inside ourselves to hide and wait to die. But why do that when there's so much living yet to do? Even if you choose to *live,* as I have, don't be surprised if some of the people who care about you don't jump on your bandwagon and vigorously cheer you on. After all, they've been gearing up for you to die, which means trying to handle their present sorrow and still reserve enough energy to get on with their own lives after you're gone.

What I'm trying to say is that dismantling the fences begins with us. Can we identify with the bystanders? Where are they coming from? Can we try to understand their emotions? No matter how it feels, it's not us patients they hate, or something we've done they're so angry about. It's AIDS.

So maybe it's time to say, "I love you," to family members or friends who are at our side, instead of waiting for them to say those words to us first. Try this: "Thanks for being with me today. Thanks for just caring." And if people come to mind who haven't been around in a while, write them a note that invites them in: "I'm sick of just thinking about dying. I need you to help me live."

There are risks in this open and honest approach, however. For one thing, the more love we invest in a relationship, the more heartbreaking it is to say "Good-bye." This perception has some validity, so it requires both patient and caregiver to reach out in faith. There is also the risk that a vulnerable request for love may be rejected. When one is already stripped naked emotionally, it hurts all the more to have somebody turn and walk away.

But these risks are worth taking. What else is more meaningful and lasting than love? Investments in people are eternal; investments in objects will just die with us. Love cannot be conquered by such a flimsy thing as AIDS. Embracing caring relationships is the only way to laugh, instead of cry, in its face.

If you're infected with HIV, broader risks are worth taking, too. For instance, reach out to try to help all those in need, whether through education or by trying to give them hope. In the world we live in, AIDS is only one of many problems. Once I got beyond self-pity, fear, and despair, and made myself available in a public sense, I discovered that many people, not just HIV-infected ones, are searching for a way to make sense of their lives. I guess they figure if I can keep going, I might know something that could help them.

It was a little surprising, but once I decided to share the values system and lessons I had learned through my illness, I didn't have to go looking for opportunities. People found me, both laypeople and medical professionals. I remember one medical student who came up after a talk I gave and said, "I thought things were tough for me, but hearing you and seeing your attitude puts my problems in a different light."

A little warning, though: Helping people is exhausting. You may have only two minutes to try to comfort a total stranger who has just told you, "I'm dying of neuroblastoma, with three months to live. Please tell me how to rise above it." He would like to have your advice condensed into five easy steps, but that's not what it's about. Handing out prescriptions like some fast-fix spiritual dispensary is useless. Instead, say—like one pilgrim telling another—"I've found some passes through the mountains of pain." Then let the other person know the route you've taken.

More importantly, I try to answer a sometimes unexpressed question: "Where does the power to traverse such awful terrain come from?" A panel was held recently in LaCrosse, and an infected young man was talking about how the power within you is the key to getting over the depression and despair. Sounds like the film *Chariots of Fire*, whose main character was a Christian with strong enough convictions to turn his back on an Olympic medal if it meant violating the Sabbath. In his sermon, he asked the question "Where does the power to run the race come from?" His answer, "From within."

But this is only a half-truth, for if the power comes from within and is of our own making, it simply does not, cannot, and will not hold up in the face of AIDS. On the other hand, there is an internal *supernatural* power available to run any race or cross any mountain, if a supernatural being lives within us (more on this in chapter 13).

While it's true that we all have a certain amount of "power," the difference between what we can produce *on our own* and what we can draw on *from an unlimited source* to face something like AIDS is the difference between trying to power a modern submarine with the most sophisticated internal combustion engine ever made instead of a nuclear reactor. You might make it out of the harbor just fine, but with time your power source would expire—and you and everybody else in the ship would perish.

Speaking of all the others in the ship, let me end this chapter with some thoughts about the people who care for HIV patients, and may be caring for you. Mark 4:35–41 NIV records an incident wherein Jesus and his disciples were crossing the lake and a "furious squall" arose. Jesus, exhausted from a long day of ministry, was sleeping in the stern. Now there's a perfect portrait of peace: power under control. But the disciples—seasoned sailors—began to fear for their lives to the point where they woke him. First Jesus rebuked the wind and spoke to the waves, "Quiet! Be still!" After all was "completely calm," he rebuked his disciples for their lack of faith.

This story shows that the power from within (the disciples' expertise) will be *inadequate* unless it is linked to the power that comes from the Lord. But my main reason for bringing it up comes from one little phrase that might be overlooked: "There were also other boats with him" (v. 36).

When we're fighting for our lives (as the disciples were), we tend to forget that the same storm is rocking the boat of many others, including family, friends, and even the larger anonymous community of mankind. As John Donne wrote, "No man is an island, entire of itself; every man is a piece of the continent, a part of the main. . . ."

The people in the other boats were just as involved, worried, and overpowered by the storm, which Jesus used to teach them where the real power comes from. This power is what we need to bear troubles so great that it feels like we're about to go under—a conviction anyone caring for an HIV-infected loved one is likely to have felt at some point, too. It may be a mother rocking her adult son, now reduced to infancy through dementia, or a father holding his dying baby girl who became HIV-infected before she was born. Perhaps it's a wife wiping her husband's brow as he shivers and shakes uncontrollably from an AIDS-related fever. Or it's the husband who holds his wife's hand as she gasps for breath in the terminal stages of *pneumocystis carinii* because she contracted AIDS in a blood transfusion.

"Dear Caregiver . . ."

If you're a caregiver for an HIV patient, you are needed far more than the patient may let on. Thank you for caring that much, when you could have simply turned away—like some have done—to get on with your own life.

Beyond reminding you of the ultimate source of your power to run, walk, or crawl through this difficult journey, I will suggest two other things that will help. First, give yourself permission to hate this disease, not the person you're caring for, or even the one who infected him or her. Perhaps you've been taught to accept all things as from the hand of God, to never question and certainly never to dispute what appears to be his will. But I think it's much healthier—emotionally, physically, and spiritually—to be positive about one's faith and negative about AIDS.

To me, AIDS seems particularly demonic. Just look at the way it works—deceiving our God-given immune system until it can no longer defend us from microscopic intruders our macrophages (cells that protect against infection) would normally gobble up. If it isn't okay to hate something this diabolical, I don't know what "righteous indignation" can possibly mean.

Second, let yourself risk loving, even if it seems like committing emotional suicide. If you really love a person with HIV infection, you will affirm that person's life instead of preparing for his or her death. The latter may seem more practical and realistic, but it certainly is callous to say, as one person said when he called to inform me of a mutual friend's death from a heart attack, "I guess you'll be joining him soon!"

"No way!" I replied. "By his stripes I *was* healed."

I plan to be around for a while, and I'm claiming life instead of resigning to death. Nobody has to tell an AIDS patient that death is a possibility. But how many are willing to say that healing is just as possible? God wants to bless his children, but we must believe and claim what he has said. If God cannot conquer AIDS, then I say, with other Christians, "Get yourself another God!"

It took a while for me to see things this way, and it was mainly through two men who risked loving me after my diagnosis became known: Ed Gungor, pastor of the church I began attending in 1990, and Glenn Klein, a friend who's been discipling me. As Glenn started reaching out to me, I told him, "You're taking a risk." He knew what I meant, that I wasn't talking about his risk of infection but something even worse—a broken heart.

"Whoa," he replied. "I know what you're saying. You and I get close, and then you die, and I'm heartbroken. But that's not going to happen. I believe you're healed."

In chapter 13, I'll tell you more about these men and what they have taught me about faith. To wrap up this chapter, I will focus on some practical ways to show your love to a person with HIV infection:

Be readily available, either in person or by phone. Sometimes your HIV-infected friend or family member will have a bad day and just needs to know that somebody cares and is there, *really* there, for him or her. If you're a Christian, what you are doing is concretely representing the Lord. Although God is the real pillar of strength, his presence and power reach out through every person who says, "I'm here for you because I love you."

Realize that saying "I love you" must imply your willingness to pay whatever price that love requires. Jesus said, "Greater love hath no man than this, that he lay down his life for his friends" (John 15:13 NIV).

I'm quite careful to whom I say these three little words, and equally selective about whom I believe when they are said to me. You can't give me a greater gift than love, but words and reality are not identical. We're either in this together or we're not. If we are, I may need you more than you can imagine. If we're not, don't lie to me, to yourself, or to God. *Be prepared to share the silence, deafening and threatening though it may be.* When you are quiet, you can enter my pain without tramping all over my soul. Trust me—you don't have to talk. You don't have to reason this through with me, though both of us may need to reason it through with God. Do you really think you can make some sense of it without separating yourself from me?

Oratory isn't needed here; fluency doesn't matter. I may be so sick and tired that I not only can't talk, but I can't listen either. I may not be able to converse intelligently, nor do I care to. So just be here with me. That's enough.

Whatever you do, don't say you know how I feel, because you can't know how I feel, even if you have AIDS yourself. Everybody is so different that no two people can possibly feel the same way, even about an experience they have shared.

Identify with me, but don't tell me all about your problems even if you hope I'll then forget my own. I have no interest in competing with you in terms of *your* pain quotient versus *mine.* Tell me some good news, please.

Keep it simple. Bring me a damp washcloth for my forehead if I'm burning up with fever, or straighten the bedding if you like, but don't fuss over me too much or I'll wonder if you're more concerned with acting concerned than whether I'm receiving what I really need.

How about reading to me, from a book or magazine or, especially, from the Bible? Almost anything will do, as long as it's not about AIDS. Or maybe you could write some letters for me. I've just been too tired lately, although every day that passes adds to my guilt at not answering my mail.

There are also many bills over on that table, but I haven't had the energy to balance my checkbook in weeks. Will you help me catch up with that?

And one other thing: Would you pull your chair right up next to my bed, and hold my hand for a while? Or perhaps just sit close and pray. Thanks. I need that more than almost anything else right now.

12

Starting Over While There's Still Time

Like any other life crisis, AIDS can be either a wedge that separates people or a powerful glue. Left alone, people can as easily be driven apart as drawn together by this illness. Without the grace of God, the marriage of Ed and Donna Rozar might be just another statistic by now, and I might still be as distant from my own kids as I was before. Instead, these relationships are stronger now than they ever were.

The simple fact is that stress of this magnitude tends to exacerbate problems that already exist, whether openly or under the surface. At first it may unify two people and their family, galvanizing and bonding them against a situation that threatens all of them. But most of us, when faced with the grinding pressure of AIDS (or cancer, Parkinson's disease, or similar debilitating illnesses), are tempted to run away, either physically or emotionally. This reaction is normal (being tempted isn't wrong in itself), and it's hard not to give in and say, "Too bad, but I'm not going to get bogged down with your problems. I've got things to do, places to go. I'm sorry you're dying, but I don't want to be part of it. So long."

To make it through this, however, we have to be realistic about how much we are willing to give, or—to turn it around—how little we are willing to give up. AIDS requires more time, energy, and personal presence of caregivers than I could possibly put into words. That's been true for us, although I haven't had some of the horrid problems others in my situation have faced.

If you're involved with AIDS, either as a patient or as a family member, your relationships are in danger, whether you realize it or not. The good news is—I'll say it again—every crisis is also an opportunity in disguise, even this one.

I have already told you how early on (when all we could think about was the process of my dying), Donna and I put our family life into overdrive, trying to cram three years of living into one year of rushing around—for the children's sake as much as for our own.

What I haven't told you yet is how things changed once I began to focus on living rather than dying, on being a father rather than being my children's memory. It didn't happen overnight, and much of it had to do with my evolving faith. But it also involved some key practical issues, like the fact that all of a sudden I had a lot more time on my hands.

When I was doing surgery, my marriage and family got the leftovers in terms of my time and energy. The long hours and constant pressure required my best efforts and my most focused attention. Lives depended on me all the time, it seemed. Even when I wasn't on call, if I was in town, how could I ignore the needs of my patients?

Since May 1989, I've gone from a secondary role as a father to understanding what being a father really is. This transition didn't happen overnight, and it wasn't always smooth; changing habits never is! My typical day is much different now, although I still go to the peripheral vascular lab four days a week to evaluate the technicians' studies and dictate my findings and recommendations.

I still get up early—5:45 A.M.—but instead of rushing off to make rounds before surgery, I wash down my medications with a drink made from aloe vera concentrate, and Sun Rider products. I haven't become a natural-foods fanatic, but I am eating smarter because I want to give my system every advantage I can.

I've cut out white sugar and flour and usually skip caffeine drinks, including coffee, tea, and colas. My sugar intake is way down, as is my consumption of red meat. But when a nutritionist said I should stay off milk products, too, I said, "Hey, I live in Cheese Land!" Nevertheless, I have learned to drink soybean milk.

When I am able I go over to the church at 6:30 A.M. for one or two hours of praise and worship, immersing myself in God's Word and especially focusing on healing Scriptures. By the time I get home, the boys are usually up, so we eat breakfast together. The girls straggle in later, unless they're going out with me for breakfast, which we do once every week or so—their choice.

Usually I get to work by 9 or 10 A.M., and stay until around noon, depending on how much dictation there is to do or if there are meetings to attend. I'm home for lunch almost every day—something that never happened before— and I return to the clinic in the early afternoon if there's still work to do.

Our favorite family time comes after supper. We play board games, Foosball, or Ping-Pong, and we read. The kids are always going to the library, so there's a book lying next to just about every chair or couch in the house. We have many family-type videos for us to watch, since network TV watching is almost nonexistent at our house.

Like me, the kids are really into computers, so we're always playing some game like "Scorched Earth," with its tanks, other weapons, and mountain peaks to shoot over. It can get pretty competitive, because whoever wins a round gets to buy more weapons. Sometimes I cheat in reverse because otherwise they get too upset and say things like, "Dad, why did you have to blow me away? You don't ever let me get a shot!"

We play checkers, and I want to learn to play chess, because Jonathan Edward and David want to play. Other times after supper, we wrestle, if I'm feeling good enough. When they all pile on me at the same time—the usual arrangement—I'll shout, "Help! You're killing me!" Sometimes I wrestle them down and yell, "Doggie pile on Jonathan Wayne (or Victoria or Christina)!" Of course, I'm protecting the victim underneath me the whole time. They like that game, but usually it's three boys against me. And the bigger they get, the harder it is to stay on top.

When it's finally time for bed, I try to leave them each night with a simple prayer. "Thank you, Lord, for another day. We trust you'll give us a good night's sleep. Thanks for watching out for our family. Thanks for being who you are."

Sometimes they'll want to be more specific, like when Jonathan Wayne prayed: "Oh, God, please make it snow tonight so we can go skiing tomorrow." In the morning there was snow on the ground, so he said, "I prayed for it! God answered my prayer." Who was I to argue with that?

Quite often I go into their rooms when the kids are asleep. I touch their heads and pray for them, "Lord, thank you for these lives, that they're part of our family. Give them wisdom and help them become godly boys and girls, men and women."

I have gone from, "Lord, I know you're going to take care of them after I'm gone," to, "Lord, I'm looking forward to seeing my grandchildren. But, Lord, give me love like yours so when I see those grandchildren, I won't be seeing my own unresolved negative stuff coming out in them."

One thing I particularly enjoy with the older kids is going out to the farm in midwinter to look at the stars. We use a computer program, "Skyglobe," to plot the heavens as they appear from our locality. It's neat to watch the kids matching the stars to the chart and getting so excited about naming the constellations—something I never shared with my own father. I have a little trouble sharing it with them, too, but only because they can pick out the formations easier than I can.

Jonathan Edward will say, "Look, Dad, there's Leo the Lion. See his front leg and his tail?" He can see it, but I need one of those cans with holes in it to see it right. That might seem impossible if you live in a city, but in midwinter in mid-Wisconsin the stars seem so clear and bright in that jet black sky that you want to try to touch them and almost believe you can.

In those "teachable moments" I remind them of the almighty God who created all this. "Look at that!" I say. "Look what he made for us. He did it for his pleasure, but also for ours, so it doesn't cost a thing to stand here and enjoy it." I don't get too preachy, but just try to flow with it. You don't have to say much to kids in times like those. God has his own way of reaching them at their level, even about these deeper things. But if I were still doing cardiac surgery, I might have missed so many opportunities to tell them what I so earnestly want them to embrace in terms of faith.

Many other teachable moments can occur because I have more time with them now, time that the older ones especially value, perhaps because they see other kids whose physician-fathers are rarely home. Jonathan Edward said once, "Dad, if you were still operating, you wouldn't be able to do all these things with us."

By contrast, sometimes our brief exchanges focus on my illness and their fears. For instance, in the late fall of 1991 Jonathan Edward said, "Dad, I sure wish you didn't have this." As I recall, that day I was physically down, and he was identifying with me. Without making light of it, I tried to explain, "Honey, it's not a perfect world. Life isn't fair." Kids understand that, I think. In their own world, little things don't always go just the way they hoped, and a minor setback becomes a tragic disappointment. Those "little things" seemed silly to me before, because, after all, I was a cardiac surgeon with more important concerns. But now that I've had some setbacks of my own, I can identify with theirs. "Let's take what we have," I say. "Deal with it and see what God is going to do. Life isn't always fair, but *he* is!"

Sometimes our interactions are humorous, like the time David came down early in the morning, saying he was too sick to make his bed or eat breakfast. In the past, because my life was so rushed, I might have ordered him to toe the line, but now I had time to play along with him a little. As an expert diagnostician, I knew his problem: CDS— computer deprivation syndrome. So I felt his head and said, as I shook mine solemnly, "Maybe you *are* a little sick. Do you think playing on the computer for a while would help you get better?"

"Sure, Dad," he replied, seriously enough that I had to fight to keep from laughing. "I think that we could eat breakfast after that."

Occasionally we overhear them talking about my illness, like when we were traveling cross-country and Jonathan Edward made some comment about "Daddy dying," and Jonathan Wayne asked, "Who's going to die? *My* daddy?" Jonathan Edward replied, "Yeah, didn't you know this sickness he has is going to cause his death?" His brother sat there, stunned, repeating, "*My* daddy?"

Donna told me that a couple of the kids have specific concerns, such as: "When Daddy dies, we want you to get married again—because we need a daddy." Obviously, our own struggle with the disease has immersed them in some pretty serious questions for children under ten.

Donna has been open and matter-of-fact with them right from the start. After all, the six of them spend so much time together, there's no way she could hide the truth even if she wanted to. Early on, she sometimes wondered how God could leave our children fatherless twice, but she still tried to field their questions truthfully and faithfully, without overwhelming them with data.

Once in home-school devotions, the verse for the day was "Ask and it shall be given; seek and ye shall find . . ." and the question to discuss was, "Have you ever asked God for anything?" Jonathan Edward became very angry. "I ask God every day to heal my daddy, and he doesn't do it." She tried to explain about God's timing, and the kinds of answers he gives, and how the fact that I was so well was an answer to our prayers.

As often as possible, Donna has used their lessons to build their courage and resolve. When they were studying history, she pointed out how the fathers of many famous people died when they were still quite young. "Remember how George Washington's father died when he was only eleven?" she said, showing them that orphaned kids don't have to be devastated for the rest of their lives.

But children can also be quite practical-minded about death and dying. Jonathan Edward once asked, "Dad, who's going to get the computers? You have to make a list now—we don't want to be arguing about that. And, Dad, have you decided about those guns? Who's going to get the .44 Magnum? I'd like that, but don't forget to write it down."

There is no doubt that although our oldest child is still only nine as I finish this, our children's view of life and their hopes and dreams have already been affected in a major way by my illness. Even though I plan to be around for thirty more years, Jonathan Edward will probably not pursue his earlier dream to be a heart surgeon like his daddy because he doesn't want to get AIDS. Now he wants to be an internist.

David, who often goes along with me to the office, loves to play doctor with my Dictaphone, imitating my reports even though he doesn't really know what they're about. He still wants to be a doctor, too, but he wants to be like me: a dictator! No longer does he want to be a belly surgeon. The reason for the change: AIDS.

I'm glad they still have some interest in medicine, but what my family needs not in the least is another *dictator*. Of all the layers of myself that AIDS has peeled away, my domineering spirit was the last to go, perhaps because it was the hardest to perceive and deal with. Thankfully, I had help, or I might have just continued being limited by this blind spot and hurting the people I love the most, especially my wife.

From my perspective, Donna and I seemed to be on different wavelengths for quite some time. I needed her more than ever before, but there just seemed to be something missing in our relationship. Sometimes this was so frustrating that I felt like splitting. If I was going to overcome this disease, I certainly didn't need strife and contention. I needed peace to be able to get on about my business and get my healing manifested. When our friction took the form of an argument, it usually centered on the idea of supernatural healing. I was contending for my life, and I tried to help her understand. Why couldn't she believe the best with me—my best, our best, our children's best? Little did I know then that our lack of a relationship was the basic problem.

Finally, Donna met with Pastor Gungor (at his urging). I prepped him for a theological dispute about supernatural healing. Instead, as they talked, Donna took the risk of telling this man, who had become one of my best friends, the truth about us. She didn't have any problem with healing; she believed that God is God, and he can do anything he wants to do. Something else was bothering her.

The real problem was that, as far as she was concerned, we didn't have a marriage—in fact, we had *never* had a marriage. From day one, my obsessive-compulsive, driven, and overbearing personality had squashed her. I had effectively quenched the possibility of our becoming "one flesh," which has to be based on mutual respect. She had stayed with me all these years not for affection, romance, security or anything else we shared or enjoyed, but simply because she felt the Lord had told her to do so.

So, it wasn't that Donna couldn't believe in my healing. Deep inside, *she didn't want me to be healed,* because AIDS had become her ticket out of a bad situation. She wasn't going to abandon me, but she wasn't about to pretend our marriage was wonderful, either.

Pastor Ed was shocked, but it wasn't until the following Wednesday that he dropped the bombshell on me. "Donna and I had a long talk last week," he began, "and as far as I can see her problem isn't with supernatural healing," he began. Then, as he looked in my eyes, friend to friend, he continued, "She *believes in it,* all right—but, she doesn't *want it* to happen to you."

My mouth dropped open. I was floored and overwhelmed with emotion at the same time. Tears came to my eyes as I wondered what he could mean. I felt like I had been kicked in the chest by a horse. My death was seen as vindication for the failure of our marriage.

"I love you, Ed," he said, "but I've only known you since the Lord's been softening your personality and building your character, partly because of your struggle with AIDS. But Donna is carrying a lot of hurt. She has a wounded spirit— and if she's told me the truth, I can't say I blame her."

"I don't think I understand," I said. "What did she say?"

"Mostly stuff about the way you've treated her and the kids—ordering everybody around, making impossible demands based on unrealistic expectations. I don't want to get in the middle of the specifics. But I couldn't believe I was hearing about the same guy sitting here in front of me. I couldn't believe you did all these things and still thought of yourself as a Christian."

"What can I do? Is it too late?" I asked.

"It's never too late," he said. "But one thing's for sure. You two need to get away, and you need to start over. You should tell her you're sorry if you hurt her, and you're willing to do anything to renew your marriage toward where it's supposed to be."

As I stood up to go, I said, "You know, it would be a lot easier just to die."

"I know it, brother," Pastor Ed replied. "It would be, but that's not what God wants for you."

I drove home, still in shock, but also relieved to finally see why we had had such conflict once I started thinking I would be healed. It was still only ten in the morning when I got home, but I asked Donna if we could talk for a few minutes. We went into the study and closed the door. Little faces did appear through the glass panes, but amazingly enough, that did not distract us.

"I'm sorry for all the hurt I've caused you," I confessed. "Pastor Ed told me some of the things you talked about, and he recommended that we get away by ourselves, spend some time alone together somewhere, and see if we can get our relationship back together. He'll find somebody to watch the kids."

Donna agreed to the plan without a lot of comment, and the following Tuesday we drove to Wausau. The Rib Mountain Inn is a nice condo-type motel. Our place came with a fireplace and kitchen. A nice, secluded setting—just what the doctor needed. We went out to eat that night, enjoying the longest and best dinner we've ever had, even when we were dating. (We've had several outings like this since then, and it has been great.)

"I want to start over if you are willing," I began. "I want us to have a marriage that reflects the plan God has for us as a couple." I don't know how I would have handled it if she had said, "Forget it!" She got pretty teary-eyed at that point, and so did I. Even though she never came right out and said yes, it was obvious that she was willing to try. We talked about the fact that it might not be easy at times, but God would sustain us through the rough spots.

After three hours at the restaurant, talking, eating, and enjoying each other's company, we returned to our room. I built a fire, and we talked for another three hours. "I need to hear your heart," I said. "Help me see what I've done wrong. Show me what it will take to have a relationship that will work."

Donna proceeded to give me a history of our marriage, from things she had struggled with to things I had done (or left undone), much that I had either forgotten or repressed. Obviously, the scars were still there for her, along with a lot of pain. "Whatever it takes to heal our marriage," I said, "I'm willing to do it. I'm contending for my life, and I need your help to win this battle."

I'm not really sure why she believed me, except perhaps she had already seen some changes taking place within me. Not that I was any kind of perfect husband yet, but she knew something was different. She decided to risk believing me— a little hesitantly at first, but far better than rejecting me. "I'm going to wait and see if this is real," she said. Fair enough, as far as I was concerned. Nobody should expect everything to change overnight because of a few words. During our encounter, one thing that Pastor Ed had told me kept popping up in my mind: "If she thinks she is right about something concerning your marriage (even though you think she may not be), she is." This advice came in handy; it was far easier to see where she was coming from by accepting as true what she said rather than trying to defend myself. Her "charges" were acknowledged as true, and I spent a lot of the time turning the other cheek. However, this is what God's love is all about. It really was not that difficult as I wanted our marriage to be healed. The Holy Spirit's prompting and restraining was the key to the success of our beginning over.

I have to thank my pastor for helping me understand about *agape* love—what it really means to love people unconditionally, to see them as God does. He values them all, even people like me who have done atrocious things. I thought when I convinced Donna to see Pastor Ed that he would fix her up and tune her in to my needs. What happened was almost exactly the opposite, one of the biggest turnabouts in *my* life. "Be forgiving and humble yourself," he had urged me. "Be more of a servant to your wife and kids." I absorbed his book, *Supernatural Relationships* and as I daily read the Bible, I began to comprehend my role as husband and father.

So now, after the rebirth of our marriage, when I'm helping by washing the clothes or the dishes or cleaning house, I'm not muttering to myself about those messy kids who are just going to clutter it up again when I turn around. Instead, I try to think about Jesus and how he got down and washed his disciples' feet—a pretty dirty job for the Son of God—without saying, "Now, guys, how about keeping these feet a little cleaner next time so my job will be easier." Sometimes I even find myself singing as I work.

I'm still far from perfect, but it's been fascinating to see how God is healing those wounds and bringing us closer together as a couple and as a family—though I must confess that being HIV-positive really gets in the way of marital intimacy!

Donna and I are much more open and spontaneous now. We sit and talk, which we never did before. I'm still pretty much a loner, so I struggle with that constantly. But I'm thankful I wasn't an active cardiac surgeon when this relationship bombshell burst, because I doubt I would have had the time or energy to really work it out.

As far as I'm concerned, experiencing this renewal has made it all worthwhile. I would rather be where I am today, with HIV infection, than where I was before, especially in terms of my marriage and family relationships. AIDS is still a curse, but God can turn even a curse around for good, if we'll just hang in there with him, trusting, believing, and growing. Becoming "one flesh," in spite of HIV, is possible because the "mystery" of that oneness relates to spirit and soul, long before it relates to the body.

I shudder to think that I could have lived to seventy-five or eighty, with Donna as my wife, practicing cardiac surgery and providing well for her and the kids, *without ever really having a marriage.* My male chauvinistic attitude prevented me from understanding the fact that even though I saw myself as head of the family, I was not really part of it. Perhaps equally devastating would have been for me to die much sooner with all these things unresolved, leaving Donna to carry it all for the rest of her life. So, either way, what has happened is better for her, as well as me. But I want you to understand that this is more a statement about God and his grace than it is about our ability to be what we know we should be.

If I hadn't had this illness, I wouldn't have had the time to really seek God, though he's been seeking me for years. I don't think I ever stopped long enough to be in fellowship with him. My prayer life was like that of many Christians—short, sweet, and superficial—unless I needed something.

Getting infected with HIV gave me the time and the hunger to be in the Word. In fact, my appetite became voracious. I have learned that there is more to being a Christian than just having a personalized ticket to heaven—invaluable as that is. The vulnerability of becoming a patient, physically, carried over into becoming God's patient, spiritually. It taught me to listen carefully to my divine Physician, hear what he had said and was still saying. If only I would repent, believe, and put my faith into action, there was much yet to be discovered in my relationship with him—a renewal of intimacy similar to, but much deeper than, what had occurred with Donna.

This deeper renewal is what I will share with you in my final chapter, hoping that you will choose a similar path in your own efforts to transform whatever difficulty you may face today into an opportunity to grow.

13

Living from the Inside Out

Once upon a time there was a Georgia lad who wanted to become a surgeon so he could stamp out disease and give sick people a better chance at life. Year after year he studied and trained, striving to perfect his skills, driven to be the best he could possibly be.

He was fast. He was good. In everything he tried, he achieved remarkable success. But something was missing. There was a barren place inside the man that neither medicine nor romance could fill—until he heard about another Healer who had brought God's Word to man.

So he believed, and was baptized, and then he turned his attention back to surgery. He thought there would be time, later, to really nurture the seed that was sprouting in his soul. But now he had more pressing things to do.

How would you make a parable of *your* life story? What lessons could it teach, especially about things you regret? The main regret I have about my life is not that I contracted HIV, but that it took the crisis of AIDS to show me I was still a baby Christian, even after all these years. My HIV

147

infection became my opportunity to grow in faith, to see realities as I never had before, to understand truths I had never heard before, and to be healed from the inside out. In effect, AIDS gave me a new lease on life.

These changes didn't happen automatically or instantaneously, as if there were a mystical magic wand to wave or a celestial button to push, through which we could control or manipulate the Almighty. We don't need to manipulate God, because he is already on our side. But if we're going to grow stronger in faith instead of weaker when testing comes, the only way to do so is to consume God's Word like a hungry baby after its mother's milk. And we have to believe all our heavenly Father's promises as deeply as a child trusts everything his earthly daddy says.

Reaching maturity of faith is a growth process, not an event, no matter what some may proclaim. Momentous perceptions and even miraculous events may be part of the process, but these only take us deeper into God's grace and truth. Every answer only leads to another more insightful question.

I have wondered how best to tell you about what I've found in terms of faith. I've tried to put myself in your place, especially if you've been walking along with me mainly because of our common interest in AIDS, but not necessarily because we share a common bond of faith.

If you are a skeptic, I wish we could talk. I would like to hear your side, and I would love to explain how I have come to see that all the questions and all the answers converged roughly two thousand years ago. An itinerant preacher-healer, who was the Son of God, was crucified on a hill called Golgotha just outside Jerusalem, not for his own sins, but to redeem all those who trust in him.

It's one thing to see yourself as a victim of an infernal disease for which there is not now a cure, nor may there ever be. I've had my own Pity Party, but good as it may feel, self-pity can change neither the past nor the future—although it quite effectively poisons the present.

Jesus of Nazareth, by contrast, was a willing victim. His horrid death was the completion, not the interruption, of his earthly task. For this purpose he had come into the world, and he steadfastly set his face to go to Jerusalem, knowing better than anyone else what would happen there. When he had fulfilled his destiny to cure something far more deadly than AIDS will ever be—the disease of sin, both in our world and as it impacts our personal lives—he said, "It is finished."

You can read the inspired account for yourself, in the Gospels. But the main reason I have invested the time and energy in telling you about my journey is because the Savior who redeemed me from the pit of hell wants to do the same for you. As far as I can see, there is no other way to generate and sustain even the *desire* to live more fully in the face of AIDS. The *ability* to do so without supernatural help does not exist in the long term, because in the long term this disease will conquer the most indomitable human spirit. The *power* to triumph in life or in death begins and ends with Jesus, because he showed by his life, death, and resurrection what knowing and trusting God is really all about.

When I first heard the news that I was HIV-positive, I had been cruising along. But after the initial shock, including the low self-esteem, depression, and confusion I've already told you about, I ended up in an emotional and spiritual limbo that lasted for months. During that period, my most intense feeling was aloneness, not just loneliness, which is more a symptom than a cause. I felt isolated, cut off from my profession, feeling like a leper in my own home, and more than a little bit forsaken by God. The illness had shaved my meager faith down to its bare foundations.

I knew from seeing hundreds of people die that we are all just passing through this world. It is not really our "home." I hoped my destination was heaven, but I wasn't very thankful about the possibility of getting there sooner than expected. But what about my destiny? During those first few months, I didn't think I had one anymore. Everywhere I looked, especially as I filled my mind with information about AIDS, everything and everybody, including me, seemed to say, "No. No. No!" This negativism nearly drowned out the "Yes. Yes. Yes!" that was coming from God.

"Yes," he spoke into our anxiety about finances—and the disability insurance was approved in just a few weeks. "Yes," he whispered as we wondered what would become of the kids—and an annuity was established to cover their education. "Yes," he murmured as I struggled with my identity and worth—and the Marshfield Clinic offered to retrain me and was actually insistent that I remain active and useful. Had I been walking by faith and not by sight, I wouldn't have needed this much proof of God's faithfulness.

It took nearly two more years of nurturing along my little faith-seedling before I realized and celebrated with the apostle Paul that ". . . no matter how many promises God has made, they are 'Yes' in Christ. And so through him the 'Amen' is spoken by us to the glory of God" (2 Cor. 1:20 NIV). His word to us is always "Yes," even when it sounds like "No."

The word *Amen* means "so let it be." It's one thing to pronounce this word at the end of a prayer that is thanking God for his faithfulness, which we did, of course, whenever we heard good news. It's totally another matter, though, to say it *and mean it* when the news is not so good, and the future seems nothing but bleak.

To put it bluntly, it seemed in those early months impossible to fulfill one of the New Testament's most difficult exhortations: "Be joyful always; pray continually; give thanks in all circumstances, for this is God's will for you in Christ Jesus" (1 Thess. 5:16–18 NIV). By myself, I never could have manufactured joy or thanksgiving, an "Amen" to God's way with me. It would have to be *his* doing; there was no doubt about that. But for me the key to letting him do this was nestled in the very next verse, "Do not put out the Spirit's fire."

For a while, deep inside me was a vague longing, like a wish you want to put on your Christmas list but hold back because you think it could never happen. I began yearning for something more, something beyond striving to set a new world record for treading water just before I drowned. If faith was worth anything, there had to be something beyond diagnosis, treatment, dying, and then being happy in heaven. Like my first experience with faith, I knew there was still something missing. Finding it took me much deeper into grace than I ever imagined possible.

Going deeper with God began in the same place it begins for everybody, in his Word. Anything else is extraneous, because only the Word of God carries the authenticity, authority, and power to cut through and expose methods, motives, defenses, distortions, and deceptions that so easily spring from the heart of man.

In March 1990 I was asked to teach the Book of Revelation in an adult Sunday school class. I wasn't sure I should accept the invitation; although I had read Revelation several times, it never meant much to me. However, I said "Yes," and again God said "Yes" to me. For nearly six months I immersed myself in this remarkable Scripture, investing at least ten hours a week in study, sometimes a lot more. For the first time in my life, I began to understand what fellowship with God is. It was an exciting, energizing, and revolutionary experience to explore God's final written word to man.

On the other hand, it was also enervating and frustrating to bring in the "pearls" I had collected week after week, only to be greeted by not much more than a yawn by many people in the class. It's entirely possible the problem was the instructor. I mean, how often can you try to express how amazing, exciting, even wild, this book of the Bible has become to you before your listeners either absorb what you're saying and get just as enthused, or simply tune you out?

Despite my frustration, the really important thing wasn't my success or failure in involving others in my quest. The quest itself was its own reward. Slowly, but surely, the Word was coming alive to me—and *in* me—as if God were right there with me, speaking it into my very soul. It didn't matter how others might respond. It only mattered how Ed Rozar responded, and he was hungry for more.

One passage in particular really arrested me and challenged me to quit straddling the fence in terms of faith:

> The Amen, the faithful and true Witness, the Beginning of the creation of God, says this: "I know your deeds, that you are neither cold nor hot; I would that you were cold or hot. So because you are lukewarm, and neither hot nor cold, I will spit you out of My mouth. Because you say, 'I am rich, and have become wealthy, and have need of nothing,' and you do not know that you are wretched and miserable and poor and blind and naked, I advise you to buy from Me gold refined by fire, that you may become rich, and white garments, that you may clothe yourself, and that the shame of your nakedness may not be revealed; and eyesalve to anoint your eyes, that you may see" (Rev. 3:14–18).

Here in words recorded near the end of the first century was a description of this cardiac surgeon near the end of the twentieth century. Before my diagnosis, faith was somewhere in the background noise of my daily existence—important, yes, but not as valuable as what I could do for myself. I didn't know how wretched, pitiful, poor, blind, and naked I was until I got that telephone call in April 1989. My destiny, as I saw it then, had been altered in less than twenty words from a guy I had never met, calling from an office I had never seen. Suddenly I was stripped bare—in more ways than I care to think about—and for a while the vulnerability and helplessness was nearly overwhelming.

But here in Revelation was an offer I couldn't refuse: gold to fill my poverty, white clothes to cover my nakedness, salve to help this blind man see. All I had to do was decide whether God was real and his promises true. Was I willing to quit straddling the fence and trust him with my whole self: spirit, soul, and body? "Amen!" I cried, and he took me deeper still. The Holy Spirit was beginning to erupt like a volcano inside me.

Before this, my whole philosophy of life was task-oriented. Life, including life in the operating room, was one unending assembly line of new challenges. When my battle with HIV began, this approach carried me forward, *at first*. We would face this with hope—and lick it if we really worked hard. But the challenge was just too big. The only way past it was through it, and the only way through it was with God in control.

So I had to quit *hoping* I would get better, because the best I could manage with that approach seemed to be turning this illness into a chronic, long-term ailment. It was like saying, "Maybe I won't be too sick too often. With his help, I will endure and try to carry on until he finally carries me into glory." I felt that approach was the same as admitting I didn't really believe that God would heal AIDS. In fact, as long as I focused on my problem with those "blind" eyes, I couldn't grasp that I could be free of this.

Real faith is more substantial—it is "being sure of what we hope for and certain of what we do not see" (Heb. 11:1 NIV). The King James Version states this even more clearly: "Now faith is the substance of things hoped for, the evidence of things not seen." Were those hoped-for things only spiritual in nature? How could anybody's faith prove things not seen?

It was time for me to cease praying in hopes of seeing some results; even this was faith mixed with doubts—lukewarm faith. Hope had me thinking, *It's going to be great when my body is free of this, when I don't have any more symptoms. My T-cells and macrophages will be reborn, and my HIV test will be negative.* Now, instead of praying about the specifics of the problem, I affirm its overall solution, which already exists in the mind and will of God. "Lord, your Word says it, and I believe it." I began reading books on healing and listening to a tape series on healing. F. F. Bosworth's *Christ the Healer* was one of the foundations from which my journey to wholeness began.

A transformation had taken place that began in my spirit. It was working itself outward to my mind, which had previously been far too cluttered with scientific facts, including symptoms, diagnosis, treatment, and prognosis. Paul describes this far better than I could: "Do not be conformed to this world, but be transformed by the renewing of your mind, that you may prove what the will of God is, that which is good and acceptable and perfect" (Rom. 12:2).

The key issue is not the renewing of our minds, though this is a formidable enough task. We are so conformed to the world's pattern that we can't even see that, until some crisis presents the opportunity to look at our values, priorities, and beliefs with different eyes. This may be doubly difficult for doctors, because the medical system forces its disciples to conform or perish.

The heart of the matter here is that only when I *am* transformed by the renewing of my mind will I be able to discern, test, approve, and contend for God's good, pleasing, and perfect will. As I see it, a slow, wasting death at an early age, leaving a wife and five children to fend for themselves, is not God's idea of Ed Rozar's destiny. If it is not his, why should it be mine?

When the Word says, "by his stripes we are healed," it's either true or it's not. If it is not, then there's nothing else to say. If it is, then we have to get past interpreting the Bible in light of our experiences. Whether we've ever seen a healing, or a demon exorcised, or another spiritual gift in operation— or even whether we think such things are possible in modern times—is not relevant to the truth of God's Word. That's going about it backward, as far as I can see.

You may believe, as I once did, that "by his stripes we are healed" is talking only about spiritual "diseases," especially the ultimate disease, spiritual death. But the way I see it now, *I am healed already*, in my spirit first, through faith in Christ and by his indwelling Spirit. But there's more, because this healing works itself outward, through my soul (including my intellect) and finally manifesting itself in my body. Just as one knows in his "knower" he is saved, I know that I *was* healed: Jesus has paid the price for me. "It" is finished.

I may not yet see scientific evidence that the HIV is gone, but I'm talking about faith—the evidence of things *not seen*. If I have to see it to believe it, what kind of "faith" is that?

Is anything too hard for God? If he can break the power of sin and destroy the works of Satan, eradicating a virus from the body of Ed Rozar should be an easy task. Shall I be a practical atheist? Shall I pray to God, but put all my hope in medicine, when modern medicine is a relatively late pretender to the throne of healing in a realm that has always been God's anyway? This virus has invaded my body from without. So, as Pastor Ed Gungor expressed it to me, "You are a prime candidate for healing."

"Hopeless" is not a word in God's vocabulary. He can do it, and it's right to trust that he will. For me and you, it is done: finished, completed. Positioning yourself to receive it is the hallmark of seeing the physical evidence of his promise. But, before I go any further, I want to make one thing perfectly clear: I'm not bragging, as if my faith is better than yours. My healing is not a divine reward for superior knowledge or actions. I'm not boasting about Ed Rozar, but about the Lord. He promises, and he delivers. We can either stand in his way, or we can believe.

We never have to beg, any more than we would expect
to beg a bank teller to let us make a withdrawal from our
bank account so we could pay the rent. If the money's in
there, we wouldn't expect the teller to say, "Ed Rozar, you're
such a braggart, thinking you can just come waltzing in here
to claim this cash."

I haven't made it yet, but, like Paul, "I press on to take
hold of that for which Christ Jesus took hold of me" (Phil.
3:12). There's nothing about me that should cause God to
do a miracle because I somehow deserve it. Then again, if it
is true that we who believe have been made "heirs of God
and joint-heirs with Christ" (Rom. 8:17 NIV), how can it be
boastful to expect our Father to do what he promises? Books
by Kenneth Hagin and Norvell Hayes helped me to drink
in the reality of God's promises to me.

I'm no saint, at least the way you may think of the word.
But the New Testament saints were generic believers who
were "holy ones" not because they acted holy; their lives
were *made* holy because they were empowered, controlled,
and filled by the Holy Spirit. We can either quench the
Spirit's fire, or we can let him ignite us. For this to happen,
we have to be open to his way.

In the middle of 1991, I started praying at the start of
each new day, "Holy Spirit, I welcome you to walk with me
this day. Lead me, guide me, fill me, use me." Gradually, as
I studied and listened and observed and prayed about it, I
came to realize that this Person, who lived within me—this
Comforter, Counselor, Helper, and Spirit of truth—held the
key to consistency and courage and power and effectiveness
for God's kingdom. Two books really helped me understand
the ministry of the Holy Spirit: Dr. Paul Cho's book *The
Holy Spirit, My Senior Partner* and Benny Hinn's *Good
Morning, Holy Spirit.*

By November I was convinced there still was something
more, something still missing that—if God wanted to give to
me—I would be a fool to resist. More than that, I began

earnestly to want everything that was within his perfect will for me. I was learning how to *unveil* this Christianity that had been part of me for seventeen years.

Years earlier, when I was part of a mission team in India, I had witnessed events that didn't correlate either with medicine as I knew it, or with rationalism as I understood it. People were healed, instantaneously and miraculously, right before our eyes. Others were released from the clutches of the Evil One and his agents, through exorcising prayer. But perhaps the most common thread tying it all together was the attitude of praise and worship, consistently marked by prophetic utterances and what is commonly called speaking in tongues.

I have to tell you, as a surgeon, I really didn't know what to think of all these things. I knew something remarkable was taking place through this group of Christian men, and I had never even imagined such stuff could happen. But, instead of studying this phenomenon until I could understand what it was about, I returned to the States and the sterile world of surgery, placing what I had witnessed on a shelf in some compartment of my mind for future reference, marked: unexplained things to pursue when you have time.

Now I had more than time. I had a need, and I had the desire to go as deep with faith as the Spirit of God was willing to take me. The result was renewal, on one level after another, until when everything else was laid bare before God, the only thing left was more fully to know him and be known by him. I wanted to love him and be loved by him to the point where we were one—at least as much as possible this side of heaven.

When it came to that, however, there were no words, at least no words I knew, that could adequately express what I wanted and needed to say. Glenn Klein began to disciple me and reach out to me like no other person short of Pastor Ed Gungor. He knew what I needed. As he is a bold messianic Jew, he would not be intimidated by a cardiac surgeon infected with HIV. One day in November 1991, we spent several hours together over lunch and then in his study at home. He preached his heart out, and then we prayed for me to receive the baptism of the Holy Spirit. The most remarkable thing happened because of that prayer and laying on of hands: From somewhere deep inside me, sounds and words I didn't understand burst forth in an experience of joyful release.

I didn't make it happen, but I believed it would, by faith. This experience was from God. Even more than that, it was God speaking to my spirit, God speaking through me. "For one who speaks in a tongue does not speak to men, but to God; for no one understands, but in his spirit he speaks mysteries"(1 Cor. 14:2).

Again, there is nothing so special about Ed Rozar that God was obligated to give me this new way of expressing the inexpressible. His only obligation is to keep his Word. While I would never say that you must have an identical experience to prove you are one of God's children, if you *are* one of his children, I recommend that you remain open to whatever gifts he wants to give you. For me, this new way of praying, which I use almost exclusively in private, has transformed my inner life almost as much as coming to Christ in the first place. The peace and joy that the filling of the Holy Spirit has brought me have been working their way from the inside out, in a healing that far exceeds everything that has happened or will happen in the future. That is surely what Job meant when he compared his earlier relationship with God to how he had come to know God more personally because of his losses: "My ears had heard of you, but now my eyes have seen you" (Job 42:5 NIV).

I know what you're thinking—not everybody is healed. This was true in Jesus' day, and it's true now. "And he did not do many miracles there because of their lack of faith" (Matt. 13:58). I don't have all the answers, but I do trust him.

People die. Sometimes they die young, and only God knows why. The answers to many such questions are not easy. But God's Word is true, regardless of what we see. His good and perfect will is what I am pursuing. Through his Spirit, he has rescued me from depression and despair. Helpless before an illness I thought spelled impending death, I had no idea that what it really spelled was *fuller life* and *more authentic faith*. Only God knew that. "Every good and perfect gift is from above, coming down from the Father of the heavenly lights, who does not change like shifting shadows" (James 1:17 NIV).

It has been quite an adventure. I wouldn't trade it for good health and mediocre faith in a million years. I know HIV will finally be eradicated from my mortal body. I have received my healing. God has a destiny for me, and I am committed to fulfilling it in his power. And when the time comes to go to my grave—as it will come for all of us eventually—I will go believing God and confessing his Word. I will not be disappointed when the time comes, for then I will finally be able to praise and worship him forever, without the hindrances that even now still come between us.

I would like to close this book with a prayer, first for myself, but then also for you:

> Father, I lay all my burdens, all my diseases, all my successes before you, at the foot of the cross. Now Lord, mold me in your will. I want to reach the destiny you have for me. I want to be able to stand before you, despite whatever illnesses, problems, or tragedies that have come into my life. I want to hear you say, "Well done, good and faithful servant."
>
> I give you myself—spirit, soul, and body—believing that your promises to me in Jesus Christ are "Yes," and only "Yes." Thank you, Lord, for being faithful. Even more, I thank you for being who you are, my

362.1
R 8932

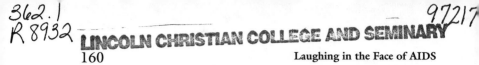
heavenly Father. You have great things in store for me, beyond what I could dare to ask or think.

Father, in Jesus' name, I pray the words on these pages would be more than words; that they would be a vehicle for your Holy Spirit, to bless, inspire, excite, and energize every person who has taken this journey with me. Amen and Amen.

3 4711 00149 7934